You

and

Your

Gut

By
Dr Peter Baratosy MBBS FACNEM

Dr Peter Baratosy is a registered Medical Doctor in Australia. He graduated from the University of Adelaide Medical School in 1978. He is a Fellow of the Australasian College of Nutritional and Environmental Medicine and is an accredited Medical Acupuncturist with the Medical Board of Australia.

Published by Dr Peter Baratosy 2024

Copyright Dr Peter Baratosy 2024

Cover Design: Nikola Boskovski

Editor: Karen Mace

ISBN - 978-0-6451053-5-3 (print version)

978-0-6451053-6-0 (eBook version)

I dedicate this book, as always, to my better half, Jenny, without whom I would not have been able to achieve writing this book. Thank you for your ongoing love, support, and encouragement.

Table of Contents

Introduction

"All disease begins in the gut."
Hippocrates (c460 BCE – c375 BCE)

A young lady presented to me in clinic with a history of having a total colectomy (removal of colon) for chronic constipation. Even after her surgery she was still complaining of bloating, bowel difficulties and not feeling well. My recommendation was to avoid all dairy and grains, as well as to use regular probiotics. At the six weeks' follow up appointment she was a different person. Her abdominal bloating was gone, her bowels were better, she had more energy and she slept better. She advised her sister, who also had chronic constipation, but still had her colon to follow the same regime. The sister made a spectacular recovery. She also told her father, who had similar symptoms, but he did not want to listen.

This story introduces the idea that there are an extra-ordinary number of people in the community who complain of some form of gastrointestinal (GI) problems. They have symptoms such as abdominal pain and cramping, bloating, a feeling of fullness, constipation, diarrhoea, or even alternating between the two, heartburn, reflux, nausea, burping and excess wind, and a vague non-specific feeling of general discomfort. Unfortunately, they are not always treated adequately, or appropriately. The above case is an extreme example but clearly shows how a GI problem should not be treated.

Whether the symptoms are mainly upper abdominal or lower abdominal, it is essential that the gut be treated as a whole.

Numerous conditions are referred to as "functional" because often when investigated, no anatomical cause can be found.

The purpose of this book is to provide information about some of the ways a functional GI problem, as well as other GI problems, can be managed. What is presented will not focus on drugs and/or surgery, but will highlight the benefits of dietary change, herbs, supplements, and nutrition. If only one person finds relief for their suffering, I will consider this book to have achieved its purpose.

Mainstream practitioners attribute many functional GI problems to a "psychological" cause because of the lack of anatomical findings. To some extent there may be a basis for this, as there is a strong relationship between the brain, the emotions, and the gut. There are also other causes that we shall discuss. However, here, I must point out that this relationship works both ways: the gut affects the brain, and the brain can affect the gut.

Rather than attempt to first treat functional GI problems psychologically, it may be more effective to begin by addressing the gut troubles, and then re-assessing to see if psychological treatment is still needed.

In my experience, many of these patients have been to their local doctor who may have referred them to a gastroenterologist. After investigations by endoscopy and/ or colonoscopy those who were told all was normal were still put on some form of pharmaceutical, either an anti-acid drug or an anti-spasmodic or in some cases, even an anti-depressant.

The diagnosis of a functional problem must be made by *exclusion* of serious pathology. Therefore, it is important to investigate. If serious pathology is found, such as an ulcer, or polyp, or inflammation, or tumour, etc. then a definite diagnosis can be made and treated appropriately.

This book provides a wholistic and functional viewpoint. I hope this will encourage people to research the matter further and then decide for themselves what their course of action will be. Modern investigation methods, such as blood tests, radiology, 'oscopies, etc., are essential so that a definitive diagnosis can be made, or at least to exclude serious pathology.

Modern medicine is focused on the western medicine paradigm which includes anatomy, physiology and pathology and the use of pharmaceuticals and surgery to treat the condition. An attempt may be made to look for causes but, in the end, generally an "anti-symptom" drug is prescribed.

Quick relief is not necessarily a cure, especially in the chronic situation. All this does is cover up the symptoms, like a band aid.

There is nothing wrong with treating the symptoms, as a doctor must make their patient comfortable and not let them suffer, however, this does not necessarily deal with the cause of the problem. It is essential to dig deeper to find the possible cause and deal with it.

Acute illnesses are usually self-limiting. Anyone can pick up a virus or infection, so an underlying cause does not necessarily need to be looked for in this situation. However, if there are recurrent attacks of the acute illness or recurrent relapses of a chronic illness, there must be a reason and this needs to be explored.

Treating recurrent acute symptoms on an

individual basis is like the game of "Whack-a-Mole". We need to look at it from a wholistic viewpoint. For example, if there is an acute attack of vomiting and diarrhoea, it is most likely that it is a viral gastroenteritis, which does get better in a few days. However, if it keeps on happening, then after the fourth or fifth time, it would be a good idea to investigate why this is recurring.

In our modern fast paced life, quick relief allows people to get back to work and play, with little thought given to any possible long-term complications. We need to deal with the underlying cause, not just relieve the symptoms.

Many patients still have symptoms after being treated by their medical practitioners. The typical story is that the doctor looked, investigated, couldn't find anything abnormal but still treated the patient with drugs of various sorts. They had excluded serious pathology, which is great, but the clinical outcome may still be unsatisfactory.

Despite the exclusion of serious pathology, patients may still have some symptoms, and they may be complaining even more because of side effects of the drugs (they are then put on more drugs to deal with side effects of the first drug). Many just do not feel well.

Sometimes doing less is more. Nature can heal; it is better to support nature to help in this process.

> *"The art of medicine consists in amusing the patient while nature cures the disease."*
> Voltaire (1694-1778)

Note: sometimes modern medicine needs to be used. Modern medicine is appropriate when the onset of the disease is acute and there is a danger of severe consequences. It can be lifesaving. The use of a natural approach is more suited to a chronic, non-life-threatening problem. There is no reason that the two cannot be used concurrently.

> *"Primum non nocere."* – *"First do no harm."*

When nothing is found, some made up name is given as a diagnosis such as "functional dyspepsia" or "irritable bowel syndrome". Or some other term, either in English – or in Latin, which is more impressive may be used. Regardless of whether the term is in English or Latin, it is basically a description of the symptoms. For example, *Proctalgia Fugax* which sounds serious, is Latin for "a fleeting pain in the backside." This does not give a basis of the condition: it is a description of the symptoms.

Why are there so many gastrointestinal problems? That is a frequently asked question. One of the main reasons is our diet. The gut is one of the first contacts with the outside world. Let me explain. Even though the gastrointestinal tract is inside the body, the lumen of the gut is still outside. From a topological* point of view, humans are like a doughnut.

* Topology - In mathematics it is the study of those properties of geometric forms that remain invariant under certain transformations, as bending or stretching.

Our diets have changed. From a genetic perspective, we are still cavemen (and cave women), we have caveman genes, caveman digestion, and caveman physiology but our diet is certainly not caveman. Also, stress has a profound effect on our gut and in this modern world to be chronically stressed has become the norm.

The modern food we eat is over processed, high in sugar, grains, trans fatty acids, chemicals, preservatives, colourings, flavouring, which are all foreign to our gut. There are antibiotics in our food, as well as the antibiotics we take, many times for trivial reasons, which can affect the symbiotic bacteria in our gut.

"Australia imports about 7 hundred tonnes of antibiotics annually. More than half of that goes into stock-feed, about 8% is for veterinary use, leaving only one-third for human use."

Dr Peter Baratosy MBBS FACNEM

(http://www.abc.net.au/science/slab/antibioics/agricuture. htm)

Antibiotics are used in the commercial production of meat. The article "Secrecy surrounding antibiotic use on farms sparks fears of superbugs" (2011) indicates how much is unknown.

"A lack of transparency on antibiotic use by the Australian farming industry is undermining efforts to prevent superbugs developing and spreading through the food supply, an infectious diseases physician and microbiologist has said."

Why are antibiotics added to animal feed?

"Livestock producers routinely give antibiotics to animals to make them grow faster or help them survive crowded, stressful, and unsanitary conditions. When these drugs are overused — by humans or animals — some bacteria become antibiotic-resistant, threatening the future effectiveness of these medicines."

(www.nrdc.org/issues/reduce-antibiotic-misuse-livestock)

What about hormones?

Alexandra Smith (Sydney Morning Herald 8 October 2011) noted that about 40% of commercial beef has added hormones but chickens have not had hormones added for the last forty years, making a mockery of supermarkets advertising "no added hormones" in their chicken products.

An update by Donna Lu (The Guardian 6 June 2021) stated that the percentage of Australia cattle that have hormones added has not changed. It remains at 40%.

An added problem is that the commercial foods we eat are grown in poor, depleted soils. Australia generally has poor soils that lack many trace minerals. Like our gut, which has a microbiome, the soil also has a microbiome, and this is depleted with the chemicals, insecticides and weedicides that are used, which in turn affects the nutritional quality of our food.

What effect does all these have on our gut? The chemicals irritate the gut. The antibiotics kill off the good bacteria and what is left are the resistant bacteria, usually pathogenic, or the yeasts, such as Candida. Then there is the stress of living in a modern dysfunctional society, which also negatively affects the gut. No wonder there are so many gastrointestinal problems today.

Whatever the gut encounters gets in through our mouths!

Some patients are satisfied because they have been

given a 'label', but we shouldn't be treating a label: we should be treating the whole person, treating the underlying cause, treating patients holistically.

Upper gastrointestinal symptoms

"A good physician treats the disease; the great physician treats the patient."
William Osler (1849-1919)

Gastrointestinal (GI) problems can be clinically divided into two categories: upper gut and lower gut.

Upper GI problems manifest, obviously, in the upper abdomen and produce symptoms such as burping, heartburn, reflux, epigastric bloating, nausea, vomiting and discomfort/pain. There is also a feeling of fullness after a few mouthfuls and/or a feeling of fullness for a long time after eating.

It must be emphasised that upper GI issues should always be considered in the context of the whole gut. The gut must be treated as a whole.

Lower GI problems present with symptoms attributed to the lower abdomen and include lower abdominal bloating, lower abdominal discomfort/pain, cramping, gurgling, diarrhoea, constipation or alternating between the two, itchy anus, passing of undigested bits of food in the faeces and excess flatulence.

To get a good history many questions need to be asked of patients about their gut and their bowels even though it may be embarrassing at times. It is important to know these things to be able to get to the bottom of the issue (sorry about the pun) in order to give appropriate treatment.

It is also very important to know what the person eats. There are certain dietary patterns that can lead to bowel problems. This will be discussed in detail later.

Even though these symptoms can be related to the upper and lower portions of the GI tract, the different parts of the GI tract influence each other, therefore the entire system should be treated wholistically.

I cannot recall the number of times I have seen patients who have tried some of the things I have recommended: they try one thing, and it doesn't work, or only minimally so they stop it and try something else which may work a little, then stop it to try something else. For a treatment to be effective, all these things should be done together, at least in the beginning, and in a coordinated fashion to support the different aspects of the gut.

In the next section we will go through these symptoms, attach significance to them, then consider what is going wrong and what can be done.

Burping

Burping is a voluntary or involuntary release of air, usually noisy, from the stomach or oesophagus. Three to four burps after a meal can be normal and is caused by releasing swallowed air. In some cultures (e.g., Japan, China) burping loudly after a meal shows appreciation for the meal and is a complement to the host/chef. When holidaying in Japan, the children followed this custom with gusto!

We all swallow air when we eat or drink. Once it gets into the gastrointestinal tract air can get out in only three ways: you can burp it out, you can release it anally and some gas will be absorbed though the gut lining and is breathed out.

A small amount of burping is normal. We all burp. Excess burping is not normal. Of course, many can voluntarily burp, and many youngsters do this on purpose to annoy their parents.

Now for some trivia!

There is a world record for the loudest burp. The Guinness Book of Records shows that Neville Sharp of Darwin, Australia set a new world record for the loudest burp registering 112.4 decibels on 29 July 2021. The loudest female burp was recorded at 107.0 decibels by

Elisa Cagnoni of Italy on the 16 June 2009.

According to the Guinness Book of Records, the longest burp was measured as 1 minute 13 seconds 57 milliseconds and was set by Michele Forgione of Italy on 16 June 2009.

Burping is only a problem if excessive. So, what can cause excess gas to enter the stomach?

Causes can be everyday events such as:

- swallowing air with eating. Fast eating: when you gulp your food down, more air is swallowed,
- gassy drinks such as soft carbonated drinks, as well as beer and champagne,
- nervousness,
- chewing gum,
- drinking with a straw,
- whipped or airy foods such as milk shakes, soufflés, etc.

Some people do bloat up, especially if they have a digestive problem. Burping may relieve some of the pressure and bring relief, albeit temporary.

Burps are not that simple. Bredenoord, Weusten, Sifrim, Timmer, and Smout (2004) compared "excess-burpers" with "normal-burpers" and found there is no difference between the two in the amount of air swallowed. The researchers also showed that there are two types of burps. One type is a gastric type i.e., the gas comes from the stomach. The other type is oesophageal i.e., the gas has not reached the stomach and comes back up from the oesophagus. The "normal burpers" only had gastric burps, while the "excess-burpers" had both gastric and oesophageal. They concluded that the "excess-burpers" brought on the burping voluntarily and therefore it was a learned behaviour.

The idea that excess burping is a learned phenomenon was demonstrated by Bredenoord, Weusten, Timmer, and Smout (2006). They showed that when excess burpers are unaware that they are being studied, or are distracted, the burping is much reduced. This points to a possible underlying psychological factor.

However, there are also medical problems that can cause excess burping. These include:

- gastro-oesophageal reflux disease (GORD),
- gall stones,
- food allergies,
- hypochlorhydria or achlorhydria,
- psychological or psychiatric conditions,
- drugs, such as narcotics, anti-diarrhoeals, and fibre supplements.

Some of these will be discussed later. However,

remember the gut should be treated as a whole and the recommendations outlined in this book are all relevant.

Dr Peter Baratosy MBBS FACNEM

Nausea and vomiting

There won't be many who read this who have never had an attack of nausea or vomiting. In fact, it is likely that everyone has been through it, either with a case of gastroenteritis, food poisoning, overeating of the Christmas turkey or perhaps that hangover. Feeling nauseous is not pleasant. You usually get over the acute attacks very quickly but imagine how distressing it would be to feel like that for weeks or months.

Nausea is defined as a sensation in the upper abdomen that gives the feeling of being about to vomit. Vomiting may not always occur, though a good vomit may relieve the symptoms of the nausea at least temporarily.

Nausea and vomiting in the acute situation are generally self-limiting. Symptoms abate within a matter of days, as long as the system is supported, with frequent small sips of fluid to prevent dehydration. Fasting helps, as does avoiding dairy. If you need something to eat, then a dry cracker or toast (though consider the gluten content) may do. If the nausea and vomiting persist for more than a few days, or become more severe, then medical advice should be obtained.

Many upper gut conditions can cause chronic nausea, and these should be investigated. Liver conditions can also cause nausea.

Nausea and vomiting in pregnancy, or morning sickness, is common. In more extreme cases, a very extreme form of nausea of pregnancy, *hyperemesis gravidarum* may occur. In such cases, there is excess vomiting to the point of dehydration, which is not good for mum or baby. Women may have to be admitted to hospital and rehydrated by continuous intravenous drip to overcome the loss of fluid. The nausea and vomiting can be so severe that in some cases, albeit rare, termination of pregnancy may be the only option. Medication may be useful but as a general principle using drugs during pregnancy should be avoided unless the benefits exceed the dangers.

In the chronic situation, nausea and vomiting is a symptom and not a disease. A good doctor will look for the underlying cause.

One cause that is often overlooked, is excess alcohol intake.

If the nausea and vomiting last for longer than two to three days without improvement, and getting worse, then a trip to the doctor or an emergency department is advisable. This is especially so for children as the main cause of death in children from nausea and vomiting is dehydration.

There are ways to treat chronic nausea. Of course,

it is important to treat the symptoms, and while doing this to look for any underlying issue.

Simple treatments include ginger (*Zingiber officinale*) which is a traditional remedy for nausea and vomiting and has been confirmed by double-blind, placebo-controlled studies (Giacosa et al., 2015; Lete & Allué, 2016).

Ginger root is readily available from most supermarkets. Cut a few rings, seep in boiling water, then cool and sip.

Another simple remedy is lemon inhalation aromatherapy. Obviously if you are vomiting, then swallowing a herb, or even a medication, may be useless as you could vomit it straight back out again. You do not need any special oils. Use a fresh lemon, scrape the skin and sniff. Important to note is that you cannot vomit up the inhaled oil (Yavari Kia, Safajou, Shahnazi, & Nazemiyeh, 2014).

Another simple remedy is peppermint (*Mentha×piperita*). You can either sip the tea, suck on a peppermint, sniff the bruised leaves of the peppermint that hopefully is growing in your back yard, or drip a few drops of peppermint oil onto a handkerchief and sniff (Tayarani-Najaran, Talasaz-Firoozi, Nasiri, Jalali, & Hassanzadeh, 2013).

The above-mentioned paper looked at using

peppermint for chemotherapy-induced nausea. If peppermint can help this severe form of nausea, it should help with other forms as well. Nausea and vomiting are major side effects of chemotherapy, and many drugs can be used to alleviate the symptoms. Unfortunately, not all work very well. Ginger has also been shown to help. See above, as well as Ryan et al. (2012).

Another natural treatment that has shown to help is acupuncture. A 2002 study by Smith, Crowther, and Beilby from Adelaide, Australia, showed that acupuncture is an effective treatment for women with nausea and retching of pregnancy.

It is important to note that during pregnancy you do not want to use drugs. The above methods are safe and have been shown to be effective. The reason I mention this study is because I was living and working in Adelaide at that time and many pregnant women with nausea came to me for acupuncture because of the publicity of this trial.

Another possibility is the use of medicinal cannabis (MC) (Parker, Rock, & Limebeer, 2011; Smith, Azariah, Lavender, Stoner, & Bettiol, 2015).

Note that MC is contra-indicated in pregnancy as CBD and THC, the two main cannabinoids, can have a negative effect on the pregnancy, as well as the foetus. This contraindication is solely based on studies of illicit cannabis smoking during pregnancy (Gesterling & Bradford, 2022).

A good principle here is, *"if in doubt – don't."*

Over the last few years, MC has become more readily available in Australia, and so doctors are now prescribing it more frequently. However, a major factor is cost as it is not cheap.

Because of the cost, and the limited number of doctors prescribing "legal MC," and because "illicit" cannabis is probably easier to obtain and cheaper, many are using cannabis obtained from unnamed sources. With "illicit" cannabis, the issue is product quality. Is it organically grown? Is it contaminated with pesticides, with heavy metals? Also, different strains of cannabis have different levels of the active ingredients. Where there is no standardization, you do not know what you are getting.

MC legislation varies from state to state and country to country, so be informed of the local laws if you decide to try cannabis.

In the context of nausea and vomiting, chronic heavy use of cannabis in the younger age group can lead to cannabinoid hyperemesis syndrome (CHS), where excess vomiting and nausea develop with cannabis use. CHS is unique as it shows the biphasic properties of cannabis; anti-nausea in low doses, while producing nausea and vomiting at high doses. The study also brought up an interesting fact that CHS was associated with hot water bathing. This was just an observation, there was no explanation (Perisetti et al., 2020).

It is important to emphasise that unregulated, chronic, heavy cannabis use in younger people can have risks. Monitored MC is generally regarded as safe.

This is an opportune time to extend the discussion on MC.

There is another system that is intimately involved in the regulation of the gut as well as many other bodily functions and that is the endocannabinoid system (ECS).

Endocannabinoid system (ECS)

Using cannabis has an action on the body because there are cannabinoid receptors in the brain and in other areas of the body. Cannabinoid receptors have a purpose, and it isn't just in case someone wants to smoke a joint.

Research has shown that our bodies make cannabinoids and that is why we have cannabis receptors. Two main receptors have been discovered, cannabis receptor 1 (CB1) and cannabis receptor 2 (CB2). CB1 receptors are neuromodulating and mostly found in the central nervous system, as well as in the lungs, liver, kidney, endocrine and reproductive organs. CB2 receptors are immunomodulating and are found in immune tissues, haemopoietic cells, throughout the circulatory system and in the digestive tract.

The body makes its own cannabinoids (endocannabinoids) and the two main cannabinoids are anandamide and 2 arachidonylglycerol (2-AG).

Research has now found that the ECS plays a major role in the regulation of the gut. The ECS is involved in motility, secretion, sensation, emesis, satiety, and inflammation (Storr & Sharkey, 2007).

Cannabis has been used since ancient times in the treatment of gastrointestinal conditions, as well as other conditions. The use of cannabis was mentioned in an ancient Egyptian text named the Ebers Papyrus (c 1550 BCE). Other ancient Egyptian texts that comment on medical cannabis are the Ramesseum III Papyrus (1700 BCE) and the Berlin papyrus (1300 BCE).

The use of cannabis to treat constipation was noted in the Chinese herbal book, Sheng-nung Pen-ts'ao Ching (神农本草经) written sometime between 200 and 250 BCE and based on an even earlier text.

In ancient India, the Sushruta Samhita (सुश्रुतसंहिता), a text compiled anywhere up to 1000 BCE (there are many opinions of the age of this text), recommended the use of cannabis as a medicine to treat diarrhoea and colic and as an appetite stimulant (marihuana "munchies"). Many ancient texts from around the world discuss the use of cannabis in many disease conditions. The use of cannabis only stopped in the 1940s when cannabis was removed from the USA pharmacopoeia and put on the banned narcotics list.

The main psychoactive component of cannabis is delta 9 tetrahydrocannabinol (THC). The other main component is the cannabidiol (CBD), commonly supplied as CBD oil, which does not contain any THC and therefore is not psychoactive.

There are ways other than use of MC to improve the ECS and the endocannabinoids:

- Cold exposure: such as a cold shower, or just washing your face in cold water can upregulate endocannabinoid levels (Krott et al., 2016).

- Use of extra virgin olive oil can upregulate CB1 tumour suppressor gene (Di Francesco et al., 2015).

- Flavonoids: a group of plant compounds found in most fruit and vegetables. Overall, the more colourful the food, the more flavonoids it contains. Other sources are chocolate (di Tomaso, Beltramo & Piomelli, 1996), tea, wine, beans, nuts, and seeds (Gertsch, Pertwee, & Di Marzo, 2010).

- Terpenes: these are highly aromatic compounds that determine the smell of many plants and herbs. One specific terpene, β caryophyllene (BCP), found in black pepper, basil, oregano, lavender, rosemary, and others, has been shown to be a CB2 agonist (Hashiesh et al., 2021).

- Kava (*Piper methysticum*) has been shown to interact with CB1 receptors (Ligresti, Villano, Allarà, Ujváry, & Di Marzo, 2012).

- Probiotics: Lactobacillus acidophilus increases the expression of CB2 receptors (Rousseaux et al., 2007).

- Stress reduction (Agrawal et al., 2012).

- Exercise. (Sparling, Giuffrida, Piomelli, Rosskopf, & Dietrich, 2003). The "runner's high" is an ECS effect, not due to endorphins as previously thought.

- Omega 3 fatty acids (McDougle et al., 2017).

- Palmitoylethanolamide (PEA) (Ahn, Johnson, & Cravatt, 2009).

- Diindolylmethane (DIM) – shown to be a partial CB 2 agonist (Yin et al., 2009).

- Sex. 2AG levels were found to be elevated on masturbation, but this could possibly relate to sexual activity in general (Fuss et al., 2017). In another study, both anandamide and 2AG were shown to be elevated in sexually aroused women (Klein, Hill, Chang, Hillard, & Gorzalka, 2012).

Some of the above points are easily adapted into a healthy lifestyle.

Palmitoylethanolamide (PEA) is an interesting substance. It is not a true cannabinoid as it cannot bind to CB1 or CB2, but one of its actions is inhibiting fatty acid amine hydrolase (FAAH), the main enzyme that breaks down anandamide, the body's main cannabinoid. So, PEA enhances the anandamide by slowing or reducing its breakdown, therefore it persists longer and has a longer lasting action (Ahn, Johnson, & Cravatt, 2009).

MC can be used for many gastrointestinal diseases including:

- chronic nausea and vomiting (MC has been used for the nausea and vomiting of chemotherapy)

- gastric ulcers

- irritable bowel syndrome (IBS)

- abdominal pain

- inflammatory bowel disease (IBD)

- colon cancer

- pancreatic cancer

- hepatic cancer

- cirrhosis

(Di Carlo & Izzo, 2003; Sreevalsan, Joseph, Jutooru, Chadalapaka, & Safe, 2011; McAllister, Soroceanu, & Desprez, 2015).

The use of MC in treating cancer continues to be controversial. However, MC can certainly be used to treat the symptoms of cancer such as pain, insomnia, and anxiety, as well as the symptoms of cancer treatment.

At present, MC, is becoming more available in Australia and the number of people being prescribed it has increased dramatically.

Unfortunately, the conventional thinking at present is to use it when "all things have failed." It shouldn't be this way.

MC is safe. No one has died from an overdose. Even the USA drug enforcement agency (DEA) has admitted that nobody has ever died of a cannabis overdose. Compare this to alcohol, a legal drug. The DEA reports at least six deaths every day due to alcohol poisoning. Thousands have died of opioid overdose. More Americans died from drug overdoses in 2016 than the number of American lives lost in the entirety of the Vietnam War, which totalled 58,200.

(https://www.cbsnews.com/news/opioids-drug-overdose-killed-more-americans-last-year-than-the-vietnam-war/ accessed 09/04/2023)

Lachenmeier and Rehm (2015) compared the risk of alcohol, tobacco, cannabis, and other illicit drugs using the margin of exposure (MOE) approach. The MOE is defined as the *"ratio between toxicological threshold (benchmark dose) and estimated human intake"*. The study showed that alcohol, nicotine, cocaine, and heroin fall into the "high risk" category with an MOE <10. The rest of the compounds fall into a "risk" category with an MOE < 100. Cannabis falls into a category on its own of an MOE >10,000!

Gable (2006) put it into another perspective with the following graph.

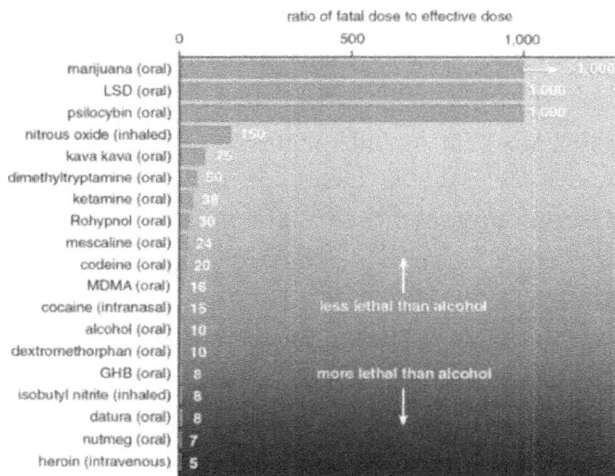

The sooner MC becomes more freely available, and cheaper, the better. More people will benefit from this exceptional herb (I consider cannabis a herb and not a drug) and have their various diseases treated safely.

First do no harm.

Other reasons for a more chronic form of nausea

are liver issues and stomach irritation. One of the symptoms of liver disease is nausea and it does not have to be overt liver failure. Even mild liver damage can cause nausea. Other symptoms can include tiredness, skin itchiness (itch without a rash), bloating, constipation, weight gain and feeling "toxic". So, if anyone presents with chronic nausea it is worth investigating the liver. For treatment of liver issues, the herb of choice is St Mary's Thistle (*Silybum marianum*).

Any stomach irritation can cause nausea, so to sooth the stomach, slippery elm bark (SEB) (*Ulmus rubra)* can be quite useful.

Dr Peter Baratosy MBBS FACNEM

Acid problems

Many people go to the doctor with heartburn, reflux or burping and burning in the epigastrium or retrosternally. There is almost an epidemic of this in today's society. Figures show that 44% of the US population suffers heartburn monthly, 14% weekly and 7% daily. That is a lot of people.

The latest figure available was that in 2015, just one brand of proton pump inhibitor (PPI), an acid suppressing drug, cost the Australian pharmaceutical benefits scheme (PBS) $229,567,718.00.

(https://www.pbs.gov.au › info › statistics › asm › asm-2015 accessed 3 May 2023)

The cost would certainly have increased since then.

As you can see, drugs for heartburn and reflux are a lucrative market.

The superficial rationale seems very simple: burning equals too much acid. Therefore, the answer is simple: neutralise or reduce acid. Neutralising or suppressing the acid stops the symptoms but does not treat the cause. It is just a band-aid solution.

Is it really that simple?

Is this really the cause of the problem?

Unfortunately, it is not.

The most common cause of heartburn is too little acid!

This may sound paradoxical, but heartburn can be caused by too little acid. Too much acid is quite rare, e.g., Zollinger-Ellison Syndrome (ZES), which occurs in one in a million people. ZES is a disease where the stomach makes too much acid due to a tumour that produces gastrin, the hormone that stimulates acid production.

To explain how too little acid can cause heartburn, it is helpful to get back to basic anatomy. The stomach is a muscular sack with a valve at the top, the gastroesophageal sphincter (GOS), also known as the lower oesophageal sphincter (LOS), and a valve at the bottom, the pyloric sphincter (PyS). Acid controls the opening and closing of these valves. The situation is more complex as there are other hormones and reflex nerve circuits involved in this, but for now I will concentrate on the acid (Holzer, 2007).

The stomach makes acid to digest food. Without acid there is no proper digestion. Stomach pH is around 1.5 to 3.5 (pH is a measure of acidity/alkalinity: low values are acidic, 7 is neutral and above 7 is alkaline). How does this work? Acid, in addition to acid sensors and reflex nerve circuits, are part of the control in the opening and closing of these valves. The whole mechanism does make sense when you consider the oesophagus is very sensitive to acid. The valve must be closed when there is acid in the stomach to prevent the acidic contents going up and burning and damaging the oesophagus (Kaye, 1979).

Conversely the valve at the bottom end of the stomach, the PyS, is also controlled by acid but in the opposite manner. When there is plenty of acid in the stomach the top valve closes, and the bottom valve is opened, so when the stomach contracts, the contents are pushed down into the duodenum. Now, in a situation where there is little or no acid, the top valve does not close properly, and the bottom valve does not open properly, so stomach contraction can push what little acid there is upwards into the oesophagus, hence the reflux and heartburn. So, you can see that any anti-acid medication will neutralise the acid, therefore no symptoms develop but this does not fix the problem.

Causes of acid reduction

Stress

We live in a stressful environment. Because of this, it is almost impossible to avoid stress, which has been shown to reduce stomach acid secretion (Esplugues et al., 1996). Our bodies respond to stress initially with the "fight and flight" response. Since digestion is not a priority when running or fighting, blood is shunted from the gut (including the stomach) to the muscles so that we can run faster and fight harder. A reduced blood flow does affect gut function.

In another study by Holtmann, Kriebel, and Singer (1990), volunteers were put under stress and gastric acid output measured. The researchers concentrated on personality traits and found that personality does have a bearing on acid production as those who scored high on 'impulsivity' had high acid output while those who scored low had low gastric acid output.

Shiraishi (1988) showed that there is a hypothalamic control of gastric acid secretion. Stress influences acid output. From a teleologic* point of view, it does make sense. During stress, fight or flight, digestion is not a priority so there is no need to make stomach acid.

*Teleology - The explanation of phenomena in terms of the purpose they serve rather than of the cause by which they arise. (English Oxford Dictionary)

Helicobacter pylori infection

Helicobacter pylori (HP) infection can also reduce stomach acid secretion. However, there are rare cases where HP increases acid and other situations where there is no change (Harris et al., 2013; Smolka & Schubert, 2017). HP will be discussed more fully later.

Ageing

In a study by Hurwitz et al. (1997), the researchers found that nearly 90% of elderly people in their study had no difficulty producing acid. However, they found only a small group of people with hypochlorhydria, and these were generally associated with atrophic gastritis.

Takahashi et al. (1993) showed a strong association between atrophic gastritis and HP.

Russell (1997) found a 30% incidence of atrophic gastritis in those older than age 60, and also showed that the prevalence increases with age.

In contrast, Britton and McLaughlin (2013) demonstrated a reduction of stomach acid production in relation to ageing.

"In the stomach, reduced fundal compliance may contribute to early satiety; however, the primary change is hypochlorhydria, which may predispose to malabsorption or bacterial overgrowth further along the GI tract."

The most common symptom of too little acid is heartburn.

So, what is the treatment?

Give more acid.

What!

Give more acid for heartburn. Well, perhaps we should heal the inflamed lower portion of the oesophagus first, if needed, with, for example, SEB. Once healed, then give the acid.

A lack of acid is called hypochlorhydria. A complete lack of acid is called achlorhydria.

Acid is essential to start the digestive process. It is needed to empty the stomach. Without acid, food will not be digested. Undigested food will rot and ferment in the intestines leading to gas production, especially hydrogen sulphide. This very smelly gas can come out of both ends as either burping or flatulence. A lack of acid produces the symptoms of bloating, food just sitting in the pit of the stomach, a feeling of fullness after only a few mouthfuls, burping and so on. Another interesting symptom is burping hours after a meal, with the smell of the food you ate hours ago still evident. Basically, the stomach has not emptied.

Acid is needed to sterilise the food as bacteria, fungi and other micro-organisms enter the body with the food. If the acid does not kill off these micro-organisms, they continue further down the gastro-intestinal tract, which has a good supply of nutrients, and they will cause trouble.

Those with hypochlorhydria do have a higher incidence of infections than those with normal stomach acid, e.g., small intestinal bacterial overgrowth (SIBO) (Dukowicz, Lacy, & Levine, 2007).

Even iatrogenic (doctor caused) hypochlorhydria caused by excess use of proton pump inhibitors (PPIs) has been shown to predispose to gut infections (Bavishi & Dupont, 2011).

Lack of acid (or an iatrogenic suppression of acid) can also lead to poor absorption of minerals and by extension, malnutrition.

Acid is needed to absorb vitamins and minerals.

Termanini et al. (1998) and Ruscin, Page, and Valuck (2002) showed that long term acid suppression interferes with B12 absorption.

Acid is needed for iron absorption. Harris et al. 2013 demonstrated that children with HP infections produce hypochlorhydria and a subsequent iron deficiency.

Sturniolo et al. (1991) and Ozutemiz, Aydin, Isler, Celik, and Batur (2002) showed that zinc absorption is also reduced by decreased gastric acidity produced by acid reducing drugs. Acid is needed to absorb zinc: zinc is needed to make acid.

Acid is needed for calcium absorption (Graziani et al., 1995).

The use of PPIs can be related to osteoporosis, and this can be related to interference with calcium absorption. Targownik et al. (2008) showed that *"Use of proton pump inhibitors for 7 or more years is associated with a significantly increased risk of an osteoporosis-related fracture."*

Andersen, Johansen, and Abrahamsen (2016) confirmed that *"New studies have further strengthened existing evidence linking use of PPIs to osteoporosis."*

This all makes sense.

Anyone with poor diet will be low in minerals. This can be compounded if they have hypochlorhydria or are taking acid suppression drugs. These people need to be monitored and supplemented.

Acid is needed to stimulate the secretion of pancreatic enzymes and the release of bile. Where there is no acid, there will be poor digestion of proteins, poor pancreatic enzyme release and therefore poor carbohydrate digestion, poor bile release and poor fat digestion. This can also lead to poor absorption of fat-soluble vitamins such as vitamins A, D and E.

There is a vicious cycle. Minerals such as zinc, vitamins such as vitamin B1, and other nutrients such as histidine, which is then converted to histamine, are needed to make the acid, yet these substances need acid to be absorbed. Catch 22!

If there is no acid, the minerals are not absorbed, and no acid can be made. Acid, therefore, needs to be supplemented. Also note that zinc is not only needed to make the acid but is also needed to make the protective mucous layer of the stomach; this is to protect the stomach from digesting itself.

If the situation is not severe the supplementation may only need to be given for a short time, the body starts to absorb the nutrients, recovers, and can start producing acid again. In other situations, the damage may-be beyond repair and in this case, supplementation may be permanent.

In mild cases digestive stimulants can be used. In the orient, herbs such as ginger are used. In the west bitters are used. Note that many of the aperitif drinks, e.g., Campari, Unicum, and Jägermeister, have a bitter taste and are traditionally used before a meal "to improve digestion." Also, who can forget the (Angostura) bitters added to gin, or to Australia's favourite drink "lemon, lime and bitters"?

Acid supplementation can be given in three main ways:

- Supplemental acid in the form of betaine HCL, which can be purchased from the health food shop. This product can be used before each meal to give more acid to the stomach and to get the digestion started.

I do not advise that you go to the pool shop and buy hydrochloric acid and drink it, although this has been done in the past. I was told by an older doctor that hydrochloric acid was on the Australian pharmaceutical benefits scheme (PBS) extemporaneous list for "digestion"; a few drops in water before each meal. Also, studies published in the 1930-50s mention the use of hydrochloric acid in the treatment of digestive symptoms (Shay & Gershan-Cohen, 1936; Rappaport, 1955).

They knew back then! Why isn't this known today? Is it because it is easier to write a script for a PPI?

It is wise to start betaine HCL with one tablet with meals, and if there is no burning and no effect, to slowly increase until there is satisfactory improvement.

- An even simpler and cheaper option is the use of apple cider vinegar (ACV). This is not hydrochloric acid, but it is an acid, containing malic acid, tartaric acid and acetic acids and can work just as well. One to two tablespoons in some water before a meal is generally all that is needed. For those who cannot tolerate the taste of the ACV, it is now available in capsules or tablets.
- Another option is lemon juice in water before each meal. Some people start the day with lemon juice in warm water but for acid replacement you should have some before each meal to improve

digestion.

Anyone with epigastric bloating, heartburn, or a feeling of fullness can try an acid supplement.

To date there have not been any peer reviewed studies done on the use of apple cider vinegar and reflux/heartburn. What I write in this book is based on personal clinical experience and anecdote, as well as the positive responses from many sites on the web. If ever they say *"There is no evidence"* this is not because the studies show it doesn't work but because there haven't yet been any studies done.

"The absence of evidence is not evidence of absence."

(Attributed to cosmologist Carl Sagan, although he was quoting another cosmologist, Martin Rees.)

Since there are no trials, we cannot say it doesn't work, especially since personal, and clinical experience show that it does work.

Do we always need double-blind studies? Some things are just plain obvious. In a tongue-in-cheek paper in the British Medical Journal (BMJ), Smith and Pell (2003), maintain that parachutes should not be used because there hasn't been a double-blind trial.

"Advocates of evidence-based medicine have criticised the adoption of interventions evaluated by using only observational data. We think that everyone might benefit if the most radical protagonists of evidence-based medicine organised and participated in a double blind, randomised, placebo controlled, crossover trial of the parachute."

Also, as one of my colleagues once said, *"You do not need a double-blind study of the effects of being run over by a bus!"*

Some things we know just work.

There is a group of people, who after trying the ACV, complain that they are worse. This can happen. These are the people who may need to be pre-treated with SEB first to heal the gut and then re-try the ACV.

Do you know anyone with an exceptionally ravenous appetite? Someone who is always hungry, may not be obese, yet have a big, bloated stomach? The problem is that the food is not digested, nutrients are poorly (or not) absorbed, so the body compensates by demanding more and more food. This partially undigested food accumulates in the colon where it starts to rot. This is followed by constipation with foul smelling flatulence, or foul diarrhoea, all caused by a lack of acid.

What about people who try to keep healthy by

swallowing vitamin pills and do not feel any better? This could be a sign of a lack of acid. Acid is needed to break apart the tablets. It is impossible to absorb the vitamins and minerals without the acid.

Unfortunately, one of the symptoms of too little acid is heartburn. This is interpreted superficially as being caused by too much acid with subsequent prescription of acid suppressors. This will aggravate the problem.

There is a huge list of diseases associated with hypochlorhydria. This is probably related to the fact that acid deficiency produces an inability to absorb nutrients. Lack of acid also interferes with proper digestion, and this causes proteins to be only partially digested into peptides (short protein chains). These peptides are then absorbed and are long enough for the body to recognise them as being a foreign protein and then react to them with an immunological response. This can lead to molecular mimicry which can be the basis for auto-immune disease.

These illnesses can be helped with nutritional supplements, as well as aiding or repairing the digestion.

The list of problems associated with poor digestion includes allergies, auto-immune diseases, thyroid diseases, diabetes mellitus, gallbladder disease, asthma, vitiligo, acne rosacea, chronic hepatitis, chronic fatigue, weak nails, dry skin, poor night vision, hypoglycaemia, weak adrenals, RA, and lupus.

In other words, any condition needs the gut and the digestion to be repaired.

Reflux

Another problem in modern western society is reflux, which is related to heartburn. Essentially, reflux is heartburn without the burning sensation. Therefore, the treatment is much the same. One of the main symptoms of reflux is burping.

Reflux can also be related to our diet.

I believe that humans were not designed to eat certain foods. I am specifically referring to grains and dairy.

In my experience a diet high in carbohydrates, especially grains, starches, and sugar, predisposes people to GORD.

I have successfully treated many patients with GORD by simply eliminating grains and sugars and putting them on a higher protein diet. The GORD improved without any other interventions.

In a series of case studies, Yancy, Provenzale, and Westman (2001) confirmed that patients with GORD who were initiated on a low carbohydrate diet experienced resolution of their GORD symptoms.

This is confirmed by the results of a more recent study, which showed that a high fat/low carbohydrate diet reduced GORD (Pointer, Rickstrew, Slaughter, Vaezi, & Silver, 2016).

<u>Case Study</u>

A gentleman consulted me with a long history of severe reflux and heartburn. He was spending a small fortune on various types of anti-acid medication which gave him only bearable relief. He had difficulty taking any acid supplements. He started on a no grain, low carbohydrate diet and the reflux and heartburn disappeared. As long as he stays on a no grain, low carbohydrate diet he is reflux free.

Digestive enzymes

The pancreas in an organ that has two basic functions:

- an endocrine function: production and release of hormones directly into the bloodstream, e.g., insulin, glucagon. This accounts for only 2% of the pancreatic mass, and
- an exocrine function: production and release of *digestive enzymes* into the duodenum to facilitate digestion. There are enzymes to digest the three main components: fats (*lipase)*, proteins (*protease)* and carbohydrates (*amylase).*

Digestive enzymes are needed to digest food properly. Without them, the food we eat would not be digested but would start to ferment and/or rot. Gases are released, which produce bloating and foul-smelling flatulence.

Maldigestion also leads to malnutrition as the nutrients cannot be absorbed.

Maldigestion also leads to foul smelling, loose faeces, full of unabsorbed fat that are difficult to flush down the toilet (steatorrhoea).

Maldigestion leads to Malabsorption and Malnutrition.

Digestive enzymes go hand in hand with stomach acid.

Pancreatic secretion consists of two components: aqueous and enzymes.

Stomach acid stimulates the duodenal mucosa to release *secretin* which then stimulates release of the pancreatic aqueous secretion.

Amino acid and fat digestion products release *cholecystokinin (CCK)* from the duodenal mucosa to stimulate release of the enzymes. CCK also influences the gall bladder to release bile.

Pancreatic insufficiency is when the pancreas cannot secrete enough enzymes to digest the food. Malabsorption occurs when there is significant decrease in enzyme secretion. Pancreatic insufficiency occurs in specific diseases such as cystic fibrosis and pancreatitis, also where there has been some surgical intervention such as gastrectomy or a pancreatic resection. It can also occur with peptic ulcers, coeliac disease (CD), Crohn's disease (CrD), and with auto-immune disease such as systemic lupus erythematosus (SLE).

These are well recognised diseases, and you must consider "pancreatic insufficiency" if treating these specific diseases. The treatment of choice is a digestive enzyme supplement.

However, there are many patients who have GI distress with non-specific signs and symptoms who cannot be categorised as having any of the above diseases.

Can we also treat these people with digestive enzymes?

If there is any evidence of malabsorption, or seeing undigested bits in the bowel action, then "yes". Although the use of acid supplementation should first be used.

Remember that acid in the duodenum stimulates the release of pancreatic enzymes.

If acid supplementation is not helping adequately, then a therapeutic trial is worth doing.

Can pancreatic insufficiency develop in the absence of these well-defined illnesses?

The answer again is "yes."

A group of patients with "dyspepsia" was investigated. One hundred and fifty-nine of these (35%) were found to have reduced exocrine pancreatic function. Out of the 159, 143 had possible or verifiable chronic pancreatitis. In about half, the diagnosis was totally unexpected (Andersen, Scheel, Rune, & Worning, 1982).

What this means is that a significant number of people with "dyspepsia" may have chronic pancreatitis and be unaware of it. Smith, Talley, Dent, Jones, and Waller (1991) found a similar situation i.e., a significant number of people with non-specific dyspepsia have chronic pancreatitis and pancreatic insufficiency without any of the classical signs. A newer study by Fujikawa et al. (2017) has confirmed these older studies.

You can have chronic pancreatitis without having any of the classical symptoms.

Note that the most common cause of chronic pancreatitis is excess alcohol intake. Gall stones are the second most common cause. Therefore, it is very important to stop (or greatly reduce) alcohol intake.

Stop drinking alcohol or greatly reduce intake.

While we are on the topic of drinking: what is

usually associated with drinking? Answer: Smoking.

Brown, as far back as 1976, showed that smoking can reduce pancreatic secretions.

Stop smoking.

To completely stop smoking and to reduce drinking to a moderate level is probably very good advice anyway.

In a group of 70 patients over age 65 who presented with malabsorption, Montgomery, Haboubi, Mike, Chesner, and Asquith (1986) discovered that 14 had pancreatic insufficiency with no history of pain, gall stones or alcoholism; 8 were found to have CD; and 15 had anatomically normal small intestines.

Other factors that can reduce pancreatic secretion and lead to malabsorption and malnourishment include:

- Age. Pancreatic exocrine secretion diminishes with age affecting men more than women. Rothenbacher et al. (2005) looked at people aged 50 years to 75 years. They found reduced pancreatic exocrine function with age. What this means is that many elderly people become malnourished, not just because of their poor diet, and reduced acid production, but also because their pancreas cannot make adequate digestive enzymes.

- Diabetes. Pancreatic insufficiency can occur in both type 1 and type 2 diabetics (Hardt et al., 2000). In addition, diabetics with a body mass index (BMI) greater than 25 (i.e., obese), may be at increased risk (Nunes et al., 2003).

- Severe protein/calorie deficiency such as in kwashiorkor and marasmus can lead to pancreatic atrophy. Two things, energy, and raw materials are needed to make enzymes (or any other protein). A severe deficiency of protein (amino acids) and calories reduces pancreatic secretion. A long-term protein/calorie deficiency can cause the pancreas to atrophy. There may be recovery but if the situation lasts too long the atrophied pancreas fibroses up and recovery is impossible (El-Hodhod, Nassar, Hetta, & Gomaa, 2005).

- Vitamin and mineral deficiency/toxicity. Vitamin and mineral deficiency would also cause problems. The rest of the body is probably not doing too well either.

There is a chicken and egg scenario here. Pancreatic insufficiency can cause malabsorption and malnutrition, but a nutritional deficiency can cause a pancreatic insufficiency.

Experiments in rats, fed on diets deficient in varying nutrients have shown pancreatic dysfunction. Deficiencies of the B complex vitamins were very prominent in producing pancreatic dysfunction.

Deficiencies in folate (Balaghi & Wagner, 1995), vitamin B2 (Gomez, Nichoalds, Singh, Simsek, & LaSure, 1988), and vitamin B3 (Singh, 1986) in rats, have produced pancreatic exocrine dysfunction.

Alcoholism is associated with vitamin B complex deficiency. This would lead to speculation that one reason for pancreatic damage caused by alcoholism is due to the vitamin B complex deficiency.

There is some evidence that a copper deficiency can cause pancreatic exocrine insufficiency. It has certainly been demonstrated to do so in rats. This seems to be more in males than females and is possibly due to the fact that oestrogen tends to promote copper retention (Fields & Lewis, 1997).

Does this occur in humans?

In one case, a person with schizophrenia was swallowing coins; over 461 USA one cent coins were found in his gastrointestinal tract. These coins were post 1981 and are composed of a zinc core with a copper coating. He developed zinc toxicity. Zinc and copper have a see-saw relationship. This patient developed a zinc toxicity, which led to a suppressed copper level. Amongst other findings in the post-mortem of this patient, pancreatic atrophy was found (Bennett et al., 1997).

Zinc deficiency can develop because of malabsorption in patients with pancreatic insufficiency (Dutta, Procaccino, & Aamodt,1998).

Vaona et al. (2005) showed that selenium is also low in patients with chronic pancreatitis.

The question is "Which came first?"

Selenium is an important antioxidant. Malabsorption can reduce selenium levels, but low selenium can increase inflammation. A vicious cycle??

- Hypertriglyceridaemia (high levels of fats (triglycerides) in the blood) is a rare cause of acute pancreatitis, and it can develop and present as a chronic pancreatitis (Yadav & Pitchumoni,

2003).

The hypertriglyceridaemia can be genetic, but it can also occur in association with diet, diabetes, pregnancy, drugs, or alcohol use.

A diet high in sugar and carbohydrates can raise triglyceride levels. It goes without saying that a high sugar and carbohydrate diet is very common in western society.

Digestive enzymes can be purchased from health food shops and some products combine acid with digestive enzymes.

Pancreatic enzymes can be obtained by prescription from your doctor and are included in the Australian pharmaceutical benefits scheme (PBS).

There are two major sources of supplemental digestive enzymes. One is from animal sources and the other from plant sources.

Pancreatic enzymes are commercially extracted from pig pancreas. The enzymes are then processed as enteric coated "micro-spheres" and encapsulated. They are so designed that the capsules dissolve in the stomach and the enteric coated "microspheres" enter the duodenum, where they break open and release the enzymes where they are needed.

Lower dose preparations can be freely purchased over the counter from health food shops, but higher dose preparations need a doctor's prescription.

Plant based enzymes such as *bromelain* (from pineapples) and *papain* (from papaya) can be substituted. These are mainly used by vegetarian patients, and in people whose religion prohibits the use of pork products.

Hopefully, by now, the rationale for using these supplements is becoming clear.

Lower gastrointestinal symptoms

"The doctor of the future will give no medicine but will interest his patient in the care of the human frame, in diet, and in the cause and prevention of disease."
Thomas A Edison (1847-1931)

As already mentioned, the symptoms of lower GI problems include lower abdominal bloating and pain, wind/flatulence, smelly flatulence, constipation and/or diarrhoea, or alternation between the two. The genesis of many of these symptoms has already been mentioned as starting higher up in the digestive tract but some are due primarily to colonic problems.

Dr Peter Baratosy MBBS FACNEM

Flatulence

No book on gastrointestinal problems would be complete without discussing flatulence, otherwise commonly known as farting. Fart is an old word, first mentioned in the 12th century. The word comes from the Old English *Feortan,* Middle English *Ferten or Farten,* which is akin to the Old High German *Ferzan* meaning "to break wind", though without the rude connotations of today.

Everybody farts! On average, the normal number of farts a day is 10. If you have more than 22 farts a day, then you do have a problem.

On average, each male fart consists of 110 millilitres of gas, while for women it is 80 millilitres, so on average males release 1.5-2.5 litres of gas a day while women release 1-1.5 litres. The difference is due mainly to women generally being smaller in size.

Now for some useless trivia. In the Guinness Book of Records, the longest fart was set by Randy Gardner in 1998, lasting 2 minutes and 49 seconds. The loudest fart record occurred in 1972 by Alvin Meshits (Yes – that is his real name!), documented as 194 decibels for one third of a second. It seems his record has not yet been broken. (Google search 2023)

Also, no one can forget Mr. Methane. He is a British flatulist or "professional farter." He has performed at the Adelaide Fringe Festival and was also on Britain's Got Talent. Check out YouTube for his interesting interpretation of the Deep Purple Classic *"Smoke on the Water."*

The main components are nitrogen, oxygen, carbon dioxide, hydrogen, and methane. All these gasses are odourless. Any odour is due to the inclusion of sulphur compounds, either from the foods we eat or from faulty bacteria digestion, fermentation, or pathogenic bacteria in the colon.

> The type of bacteria in the colon can influence the amount and odour of the flatulence.

Other sources of gas are:

- swallowing excess air when we eat, especially if we eat fast,
- carbonated beverages,
- drinking with a straw,
- chewing gum,
- talking too much.

Note that the same causes are mentioned with burping. Obviously if you do not release the gas through burping, they will be either absorbed through the gut and breathed out or released anally.

Foods that cause the most gas are carbohydrates and the carbohydrate that is the worst offender, as anyone who has seen the film *"Blazing Saddles"* knows, is beans. Other foods include broccoli, brussels sprouts, cabbage, and cauliflower. It is interesting to note that many of the foods that are considered healthy are the ones producing the most gas.

Treatment for excess flatulence includes:

- changing the diet, removing excess sugars and carbohydrates (which is healthy in itself),
- improving the digestion, so that the food is digested and not fermented in the gut, and
- removing "bad" bacteria and micro-organisms from the gut and replacing them with "good" bacteria.

As well we should avoid all the above factors which promote excess gas swallowing.

Constipation and diarrhoea

Before we start discussing constipation and diarrhea, we must devise a method to categorize the bowel motions. This can be useful in history taking and with follow up. The standard method is with the use of the Bristol Stool Chart, based on a study by Lewis and Heaton in 1997. Most of my patients have a giggle when they see this, or they tell me they have seen this on the inside of the toilet door at a friend's place.

Bristol Stool Chart – appendix 1

As part of my history taking, I ask many questions about bowel actions. I ask, not only about the physical characteristics as depicted on the Bristol Stool Chart, but colour as well, and, if there is blood, mucous or any obvious undigested bits seen. It is surprising that many have difficulty answering these questions. Many just do not look. Some are quite embarrassed, but these questions *must* be asked, otherwise a diagnosis may be missed.

Bowel motion colour can also tell us a lot. Up till recently when I asked about bowel colour, I had to point to various shades of brown from around the office, but this changed after looking for paint in the hardware shop. While I was looking at the colour chart to choose a colour, it dawned on me; why not use a paint colour chart for bowel motion colour? I found a chart with various brown colours and now I use that. The chart has light to medium to dark brown, each with a colour name, which I record in the notes. If the colour is not on the chart, then there is definitely a problem!

A normal bowel colour is a dark brown, the colour coming mainly from bile. A light-coloured bowel action reflects reduced bile production.

Constipation

"Constipation is an acute or chronic condition in which bowel movements occur less often than usual or consist of hard, dry stools that are painful or difficult to pass. Bowel habits vary, but an adult who has not had a bowel movement in three days, or a child who has not had a bowel movement in four days is considered constipated."
(https://medicaldictionary.thefreedictionary.com/constipation accessed 11 April 2023)

From this you can see that constipation does not refer just to a frequency problem but also to the consistency of the faeces themselves and any difficulty in passing the motion. The average number of bowel movements is three a day to once every three days, although, as stated above, the condition of the faeces must also be considered.

The first important thing to say about constipation is that it is a symptom, not a disease.

Constipation is a symptom not a disease.

Constipation is a very common problem. Almost everyone gets constipated occasionally, but it generally resolves spontaneously.

It is, in fact, the most common gastrointestinal complaint in the USA, and accounts for about 2.5 million doctor visits annually. This figure is based on a study by Arce, Ermocilla, and Costa (2002). Probably by now the numbers would be much higher. However, rather than bothering to spend money to see a doctor, many buy over-the-counter laxatives, spending millions of dollars every year. In 2019, more than US $1.5 billion were spent on over the counter laxatives (Rao & Brenner, 2021).

If constipation is a symptom and not a disease, what are the underlying causes?

These can be many and varied and include:

- diet, e.g., dairy allergy or intolerance,
- lack of fibre in diet, e.g., excessively refined diet,
- poor fluid intake,
- lack of bile production,
- lack of exercise,
- medications, e.g., analgesics, opioids,
- IBS,
- laxative abuse,

- ignoring urge, e.g., working conditions,
- specific bowel diseases, e.g., coeliac disease (CD), colon cancer,
- neurological problems, e.g., stroke, paraplegia, MS. Constipation can also be a prodrome to Parkinson's disease (PD).
- specific diseases, e.g., hypothyroidism, diabetes,
- painful rectal conditions, e.g., haemorrhoids, anal fissure,
- changes in routine, e.g., travelling,
- life changes, e.g., pregnancy, old age,
- psychological/psychiatric, e.g., excess concern with bowels.

Diagnosis can be made on taking a detailed history, physical examination, including a digital rectal examination and simple investigations including blood tests, sigmoidoscopy, and colonoscopy or barium x-ray examination. Most causes are obvious. However, it can be difficult to treat patients in situations where no obvious cause can be found. Once any physical cause is excluded, then the most common cause is probably the diet. A high fibre diet should be encouraged, especially in the form of vegetables, salads, and some fruits. Adequate water intake is important. It is important to note however, that if your fluid intake is low, then drinking more would help. If, you already drink adequate water, then drinking more will not help the constipation.

Extra fibre can be given in the form of psyllium husks. Wheat bran, or any other grain, should be discouraged because of the possibility of gluten intolerance.

The use of a specific probiotic, Escherichia coli Nissle 1917 (EcN), has been shown to treat chronic constipation. The story goes that in 1917, during World War 1, when many soldiers came down with dysentery and other intestinal diseases, there was one soldier who did not develop any gastrointestinal problems at all. Professor Alfred Nissle isolated one strain of E. coli from this soldier. He then perpetuated the strain which has been extensively studied since. You often hear of gastric epidemics caused by E. coli; if you do, don't worry as this is a non-pathogenic form of E. coli. E. coli is a normal commensal in the gut.

EcN has been shown by Bruckschen and Horosiewicz (1994) and Mollenbrink and Bruckschen (1994) to be very useful in chronic constipation. Although these studies were done some time ago, they are still valid.

Newer studies have shown EcN to have a broader effect on the gut.

Sonnenborn and Schulze (2009) wrote, "*The restoration of a disturbed gut barrier by EcN is thought to be due to the stimulation of epithelial defensin production as well as to a 'sealing effect' on the tight junctions of the enterocytes. EcN has also been shown to induce the development of the gut immune system in animal models and human newborns. In addition, it has been found that products of EcN metabolism, probably acetic acid, promote colonic motility that might be helpful for therapeutic application in chronically constipated patients. Randomized controlled clinical trials (RCTs) have shown EcN to be therapeutically effective in rather diverse indications, such as ulcerative colitis, chronic constipation, and acute and protracted diarrhea."*

Another very common cause of constipation, especially in children, is dairy allergy or intolerance. Most people seem to think that a dairy allergy/intolerance can only cause diarrhoea, however, as shown by Iacono et al. (1998) and Daher et al. (2001), dairy allergy/intolerance can also cause constipation, and this can occur not only in children, but also in adults.

Case Study

A 75-year-old lady consulted me with a history of, as she put it, a "lifelong history of constipation." She was an avid milk drinker. My suggestion was to stop dairy. Within two weeks her "lifelong constipation" had virtually disappeared.

Dr Peter Baratosy MBBS FACNEM

Diarrhoea

*"Diarrhoea is defined as the frequent passage
of loose or watery stools."*
(Murtagh,1992)

We can classify diarrhoea into two categories: acute, defined as diarrhoea lasting less than two weeks, and chronic, defined as diarrhoea lasting longer than two weeks.

Acute diarrhoea is very common and most everyone would have had a dose sometime in their life. It is usually caused by bacteria or a virus or by some toxin in food.

Food poisoning and viral gastroenteritis are generally self-limiting.

In the well-nourished population, diarrhoea is considered a minor illness, although in under-developed countries, where malnutrition is rife, it can be a very dangerous condition. According to the World Health Organization (WHO), *"Diarrhoeal disease is the second leading cause of death in children under five years old and is responsible for killing around 525,000 children every year."*

(https://www.who.int › news-room › fact-sheets › detail › diarrhoeal-disease accessed 27 June 2023)

Chronic diarrhoea is not a disease, rather it is usually a symptom of some underlying disease, such as:

- irritable bowel syndrome (IBS),
- small intestinal bacterial overgrowth (SIBO),
- intestinal infections, e.g., Giardia, Blastocystis, Dientamoeba fragilis, Salmonella, cholera, etc.,
- Crohn's disease (CrD),
- Ulcerative colitis (UC),
- lactose intolerance,
- CD,
- gluten intolerance,
- inappropriate diet,
- laxative abuse,
- systemic disease, hyperthyroidism, diabetes,
- food allergies/intolerances,
- spurious diarrhoea. This is in fact a case of constipation where the bowel is so blocked up that the only thing that can be passed are the liquid bowel contents from higher up in the colon. The treatment for this type of diarrhoea is an enema.

> Chronic diarrhoea is a symptom not a disease.

In the acute phase, treatment is supportive, especially fluid replacement. Generally oral fluid and mineral replacement is adequate but if there is severe vomiting or extreme dehydration, then intravenous fluid replacement is needed. Giving anti-diarrhoeal agents is not recommended as diarrhoea is the body's way of getting rid of toxins. Plugging up the bowel interferes with the self-cleaning mechanism. This does not mean that anti-diarrhoeal medications should never be used. There are times such as travelling when they can be very useful, but they should only ever be used for a limited time.

Allen, Okoko, Martinez, Gregorio, and Dans (2004) showed that probiotics can reduce the severity and length of diarrhoeal illness. However, in a newer study carried out in 2020, Collinson et al. concluded that they really weren't sure that probiotics did reduce the length and severity of diarrhoea. However, as there may be some limited benefit, it is always worth trying.

From personal experience, probiotics can also be used to prevent traveller's diarrhoea. On a trip to Bali, the whole group developed "Bali Belly" except for me. I was the only one taking probiotics.

Probiotics, according to Guo, Goldenberg,

Humphrey, El Dib, and Johnston (2019), can prevent paediatric antibiotic associated diarrhoea.

Zinc supplementation has also been shown to be useful in treating diarrhoea. Dutta et al. (2000) demonstrated that it can be effective, cheap and lifesaving especially in malnourished children.

Chronic diarrhoea is different. The underlying cause must be found and treated. Following is a discussion of many conditions that often cause chronic diarrhoea.

Dr Peter Baratosy MBBS FACNEM

Lactose intolerance

Lactose intolerance is a condition where the sugar, lactose, cannot be digested because of the lack of a specific enzyme, *lactase*. This may be due to a congenital lack of the enzyme, as occurs in many ethnic and racial groups or it may be due to a bowel injury, such as severe gastroenteritis. In this latter case, the lactose intolerance is only temporary. This is a good reason not to drink milk after a gastroenteritis.

Up to 75% of African Americans and American Indians and 90% of Asian Americans are lactose intolerant. In the USA this would amount to approximately 50 million people. The condition is the least evident amongst those with Northern European descendants.

Some are born with a total lactase deficiency, and some develop it slowly after the age of two years. After this age the gut produces less lactase. We could speculate here. The body stops making the enzyme. Could this be an inborn programme indicating that after that age we do not have to, or need to, drink milk, as lactose is the main sugar of milk?

Symptoms of lactose intolerance include nausea, cramps, bloating, diarrhoea, and flatulence. It generally does not cause burping. Symptoms start approximately thirty minutes to two hours after ingesting lactose. Severity varies between individuals and depends on levels of residual lactase present.

The condition can be suspected by the history and confirmed by a hydrogen breath test. This test measures the amount of hydrogen in the breath. Normally it is very low but bacteria in the gut ferment undigested lactose producing hydrogen, amongst other gases.

Another simple test is the stool acidity test. Undigested lactose fermented by gut bacteria produces lactic acid and other short chained fatty acids thus making the stools more acidic. Treatment is simple: do not drink milk. It is not an essential food for humans.

I maintain that cow's milk is only good for baby cows. Even then, after a month or so, the calf must start to eat grass for the magnesium content, as there is little magnesium in the milk. Humans do not need to drink milk after weaning off mother's breast milk. They do not need the mammary secretions from another species.

Of course, there are many who can drink milk and eat dairy products such as cheese and ice cream without issue. There are also many who can eat gluten without issue. My advice regarding dairy and gluten avoidance is for people with gut problems.

"If it ain't broke, don't fix it!"

Another treatment is to supplement lactase tablets, but it is preferable to simply stop drinking milk.

Lactose is a common ingredient in many pharmaceutical tablets. One patient couldn't take her medication because of the lactose, so she took the lactase tablets before she took the pharmaceutical.

In this next section, I will discuss the difference between Lactose Intolerance, Milk Allergy and Milk Intolerance.

- Lactose intolerance is an inability to digest the sugar of milk due to the lack of the enzyme lactase.
- Milk allergy is an actual allergy to milk, especially the milk proteins. Milk antibodies can be detected, and skin allergy prick tests are positive. This is relatively uncommon.
- Milk intolerance is where there is no allergy but there is an undefined, non-immunologic sensitivity to the milk protein. These distinctions are important to bear in mind as we continue.

A1 milk vs A2 milk

If you really want to drink milk, then it is worth trying A2 milk. A2 milk is milk from certain breeds of cows. Be aware that there are some misleading statements on some of the milk cartons. Some say, "contains A1 and A2 proteins". This is not good enough. If you want to drink A2 milk it should be certified completely A2 milk. The milk protein, casein, is designated as A1 and A2. A2 is the natural form of the casein protein. Sheep, goats, camel, even human milk is A2. A1 is the mutation, and the difference is only 1 amino acid at position 67, where there is histidine, while in A2 there is a proline. This one alteration makes a difference; it changes the shape the protein folds into, and shape is related to function. With this change in shape, when A1 is broken down, a peptide called *beta-casomorphine-7* (BCM-7) is created and this peptide has opioid properties. Opioids are known to have effects on the gut, e.g., constipation and on the brain, e.g., "brain fog". This can influence a proportion of the population. A1 milk consumption does cause increased gut issues in some, compared to A2 milk (Ho, Woodford, Kukuljan, & Pal, 2014).

A2 is the milk from the small Jersey house cow. It is possible that it may cause fewer problems for those who have a dairy intolerance. Jianqin et al. (2016) wrote,

Dr Peter Baratosy MBBS FACNEM

"Consumption of milk containing A1 β-casein was associated with increased gastrointestinal inflammation, worsening of PD3 (Post Dairy Digestive Discomfort) symptoms, delayed transit, and decreased cognitive processing speed and accuracy. Because elimination of A1 β-casein attenuated these effects, some symptoms of lactose intolerance may stem from inflammation it triggers and can be avoided by consuming milk containing only the A2 type of beta casein."

Irritable bowel syndrome (IBS)

This is probably the most common diagnosis encountered and you may be wondering why I have not discussed it to any extent.

Sherlock Holmes once observed that you may notice a thing more by its absence, than by its presence: that is, the vital clue is what is NOT there, rather than what is there.

You are right, how observant you are! I have not discussed IBS to a great degree because, in reality, a large portion of this whole book is about IBS.

IBS is a functional gut problem that cannot be explained by standard theory and is pigeonholed under the name of IBS. The name, however, is a description of the symptoms rather than a description of what IBS is.

Fortunately, there is an answer. I think the main cause of IBS is a combination of some, or all, of the conditions that are discussed in this book, namely: acid deficiency, pancreatic enzyme deficiency, food intolerance, (especially grains (gluten) or dairy), dysbiosis, small intestinal bacterial overgrowth (SIBO) and leaky gut syndrome (LGS).

SIBO – Small intestinal bacterial overgrowth

"If you have a rock in your shoe and it's making your foot hurt the conventional approach would be to give you a diagnosis of foot pain, (Pedalgia sounds better – the author) and a prescription for an analgesic to reduce the pain. Certainly, it would help, but in functional medicine, we take off your shoe and dump out the rock."

Chris Kresser (California Centre for Functional Medicine)

SIBO can be defined as *"Excessive concentrations of colonic bacteria (exceeding 100,000 microorganisms per mL) within the duodenum or jejunum. SIBO may produce abdominal pain, bloating, and diarrhea owing to malabsorption."* (Medical Dictionary, © 2009 Farlex and Partners)

It is important to note at this point that there generally are little or no bacteria in the small intestine (SI).

SIBO then, is a condition where there is an overgrowth of bacteria in the SI, and this causes a variety of symptoms including bloating, pain, diarrhoea, or constipation. This description sounds just like IBS. Is there a difference? Can we differentiate SIBO from IBS? Or is it the same thing? Is it a subset of IBS? These are some interesting questions. Ghoshal, Shukla, and Ghoshal (2017) showed that a substantial proportion of people with IBS actually have SIBO. This study reported that up to 78% of IBS is actually SIBO. The range went from 4% to 78%, while in controls the range was from 1% to 40%.

Why such a big range? Possibly it is because it is a new concept and because diagnosing is difficult. However, as we progress, diagnosis is becoming easier as Dukowicz, Lacy, and Levine (2007) wrote, *"This apparent increase in prevalence may have occurred, in part, because readily available diagnostic tests have improved our ability to diagnose SIBO."*

How to test for SIBO?

There are no perfect tests to diagnose SIBO. The most direct way, which is also technically near impossible is to obtain a sample of small intestine contents.

There is an easier method, a breath test. After swallowing a non-absorbable sugar solution, the patient blows into a bag to collect the air. This is done every twenty to thirty minutes (depending on the protocol) for up to three hours. Once the sugar solution reaches the SI, the bacteria there metabolises and releases hydrogen and methane. Only bacteria produce hydrogen and methane. Human cells cannot produce these gasses. The gasses diffuse into the blood stream then out into the lungs. It takes about two hours for the sugar solution to reach the SI, so if there is a rise in methane and hydrogen at the two-hour mark, then the assumption is that bacteria are there.

Normally there are no bacteria in the SI. The difficulty is in the interpretation of the results. What is positive to some is negative to others. As stated earlier there are no perfect tests. This would also account for the large variation in the incidence of SIBO. However, in 2017 a consensus was reached, so studies after 2017 may be more accurate (Rezaie et al., 2017).

What predisposes to SIBO?

SIBO develops when the normal homeostatic mechanisms of the gut fail for whatever reason. There are many processes that fail but to keep it simple only three will be discussed:

- gastric acid deficiency,
- alteration of intestinal motility, and
- ileocaecal valve (ICV) dysfunction.

Gastric acid is essential in suppressing/killing off bacteria that enter the stomach and therefore stops it passing further into the SI. Hypochlorhydria (low stomach acid) can be a part of ageing but can also be iatrogenic, or doctor caused. As stated earlier in this book, one of the most frequently prescribed drugs is the family of acid suppressing drugs to treat heartburn. Earlier discussion has shown that many cases of heartburn are not due to too much acid but too little acid. Compare et al. (2011) and Lombardo, Foti, Ruggia, and Chiecchio (2010) demonstrated that the use of acid-suppressing drugs can predispose to SIBO.

Any abnormality in the smooth functioning of the SI motility can predispose to SIBO. There are many causes for this, including:

- chronic renal failure which can cause neuropathic damage to the gut nerves,
- neuropathic processes – diabetes,
- myopathic diseases, such as scleroderma,
- structural abnormalities of the GI tract, surgery, bypasses, adhesions, etc. So here again this could be an iatrogenic disease,
- defective immune function,
- CD,
- gall bladder disease,
- hypothyroidism.

Probably one of the most common predisposing factors is gall bladder disease. Bile has many functions:

- Bile is a fat emulsifier, that is it acts as a "soap" to "wash" away the bacteria in the SI.
- Bile has an antimicrobial effect.
- Bile can seal up the leaky gut.
- Bile alters SI motility, slowing it down. Conversely, bile can increase large intestine motility. Bile does this by regulating the "migrating motor complex" which is the ability of the intestines to move what you've eaten-to clean up the bowels.

- Bile promotes commensal bacteria and inhibits pathogenic bacteria.

As shown above, proper gall bladder function is essential and is important in the prevention of SIBO.

Does gall bladder removal (cholecystectomy) predispose to SIBO? Various studies have resulted in different conclusions. Sung et al. (2015) and Kim et al. (2017) say "yes".

However, Gabbard, Lacy, Levine, and Crowell (2014) showed no association. More recently, Kim, Paik, Song, Kim, and Lee (2018) showed that gall stones are associated with SIBO, but not necessarily with cholecystectomy.

The evidence so far indicates that the issue is probably related to the reduced bile flow. This is most likely due to gall stones, rather than the removal of the gall bladder *per se*, as bile still flows after a cholecystectomy although as a continuous drip rather than in bursts. However, if SIBO symptoms do develop, then they can still be treated with, e.g., dandelion (*Taraxacum officinale)*, which is an herb to increase bile flow, or with ox bile supplements.

Ileocaecal valve (ICV) dysfunction has been implicated in SIBO. The ICV is a one-way valve between the sterile SI and the bacteria filled large intestine (LI). This one-way valve allows "food" (for simplicity I will use the word "food" here, although it is partially digested food remnants) to move periodically from the SI to LI or colon, for further processing. Problems can occur if the valve is disturbed. If the valve is incompetent, i.e., stuck open, then bacteria can migrate up into the SI. Evidence suggests, then, that an incompetent ICV can predispose to SIBO (Roland et al., 2014; Chandler Roland et al., 2017).

Also, a chronically open ICV can allow partly processed food to continually enter the LI and lead to diarrhoea. Conversely, a chronically shut ICV will prevent the food in the SI from entering the LI, the food remains in the SI and starts to rot, it then ferments, which leads to bloating, bad breath, toxicity etc. The ICV dysfunction is now only just being recognised by the mainstream, but integrative and functional medical doctors have known about this condition for some time.

Despite what I have just said, a new study has cast doubts on some of those above-mentioned predisposing factors for developing SIBO. Brechmann, Sperlbaum, and Schmiegel (2017) showed a significant association with SIBO and impairment of gastric acid barrier (gastrectomy), impairment of intestinal clearance (gastric surgery, colonic resection, stenosis, gastroparesis, neuropathy), immunological factors (drug induced immune suppression), hypothyroidism and diabetes. The strongest predictors were gastric surgery, stenoses, medical immunosuppression and levothyroxine replacement (hypothyroidism).

This study did <u>not</u> show any association with any abdominal surgery, cholecystectomy, ileocaecal resection, vagotomy or IgA deficiency. The study also showed that a past history of appendicectomy seemed to reduce the risk of SIBO. There was no explanation as to why. The researchers did conclude that there may be some bias because the population of patients studied consisted mainly of inpatients and the study was retrospective, which led to certain limitations.

The surprising finding was that ileocaecal resection did not predispose to SIBO, while other studies of ICV dysfunction did show a correlation.

While speaking about the appendix, for years it was regarded as an "evolutionary vestige", an organ with no function, except to become inflamed, thus requiring surgical removal. However, Salminen et al. in 2015, demonstrated that uncomplicated appendicitis can be treated with antibiotics, preventing the need for surgery.

It is interesting to note that only a few mammals other than humans have an appendix. Randal Bollinger, Barbas, Bush, Lin, and Parker (2007) demonstrated that the appendix does have an important function. The appendix can possibly be a "safe house" for gut commensal bacteria, providing support for reinoculating the gut after some catastrophic event, as well as having a relationship to biofilms in the large intestine.

Back to the ICV!

The ICV is under the control of the digestive system, the nervous system, and also under hormonal control.

There are a number of foods that can irritate the ICV such as wheat, corn (especially popcorn), milk, soy, potato crisps, nuts, seeds, whole grains, spicy foods, chocolate, alcohol, and caffeine. Also, some high roughage foods, despite being considered healthy, can, for some with a gut problem, make matters worse. So, it would be a good idea to reduce some of these foods for a matter of two to three weeks and re-assess.

The ICV is under the control of the autonomic nervous system (ANS); the sympathetic nervous system (SNS) and the para sympathetic nervous system (PNS). They are closely related to the stress response as the SNS is associated with the fight and flight response, while the PNS is associated with the rest, digest, reproduce state, the ideal state for us to be in most of the time. In a stress situation (and who in this modern world is not stressed?) the SNS is activated; this has the effect of shutting the ICV, preventing waste from getting out and trapping it in the small intestines leading to bloating, bad breath, and toxicity, etc. In the adrenal burnout/chronic fatigue scenario, the PNS is more dominant, leading to the ICV being stuck in the open position, which prevents proper nutrient absorption from the SI and allows bacteria to move backwards into the SI to produce a SIBO. Not a good scenario.

Hormones, such as cortisol can have a negative effect, and this leads to a situation where the stresses in today's society can result in gut problems. Stress, and the negative emotions associated with it, such as worry, play a huge role in gut dysfunction, including ICV dysfunction. The connection between stress and the gut has been discussed simply because stress is a cause of so much GI distress. Stress is possibly the biggest health issue of this century.

Which eating plan is best for IBS and SIBO?

What about IBS and SIBO? What would be the best diet? As the word "diet" often has negative connotations, I prefer to use the term "eating pattern". The suggestion is to follow a low FODMAP (another of the latest "buzz" words) eating pattern. The FODMAP eating pattern is based on research from the Monash University in Australia. The researchers look at what foods can aggravate IBS and by extension, SIBO, as a large proportion of IBS is SIBO.

What are FODMAPs?

FODMAPs are short chained carbohydrates that are poorly absorbed in the small intestine. FODMAP stands for **F**ermentable, **O**ligosaccharides, **D**isaccharides, **M**onosaccharides **A**nd **P**olyols. These carbohydrates are poorly absorbed in the small intestine and water is osmotically drawn in leading to diarrhoea. These carbohydrates travel to the large intestine where they are fermented. The gas that is produced leads to symptoms of bloating, flatulence, constipation, pain, and nausea. These symptoms can be quite distressing. They often result in anxiety and stress, which greatly interfere with normal everyday living. As we have seen, many people, an estimated 1 in 7, suffer from gut issues. The research has shown that the low FODMAP diet can help three out of four with this problem. However, it is not a cure. You cannot stay on the low FODMAP diet indefinitely. This eating pattern can best be described as:

- a diagnostic tool, and
- short term temporary treatment for anything from two to six weeks at a time.

The low FODMAP eating pattern alleviates the symptoms: it does not cure. These foods are not the cause of the IBS/SIBO. I recommend that, to help heal the gut, you follow this eating pattern while doing the other things mentioned in this book. Once you start to feel better you can begin to introduce these foods, slowly, and one at a time. If a food continues to aggravate you, then don't eat it! Although you can research FODMAPS on the internet, getting help from a nutritional doctor or a dietician can be more useful. Another source of information is the Monash University FODMAP app for your smart phone, it is a free download.

List of high FODMAP foods to avoid

- some vegetables. Especially onions, and garlic
- fruits, particularly "stone" fruits like peaches and apricots
- dried fruits and fruit juice concentrate
- beans and lentils
- wheat and rye. Breads, pasta, cereals
- dairy products that contain lactose, such as milk and ice cream
- nuts, including cashews and pistachios
- sweeteners and artificial sweeteners

If you choose to further investigate this eating pattern, you will note that it eliminates dairy, grains, gluten and sugars which, as stated in this book, is a healthy thing to do anyway.

How is SIBO treated?

Dukowicz, Lacy, and Levine (2007) state that the three goals of SIBO treatment are to:

- correct the underlying cause,
- provide nutritional support, and
- treat the overgrowth.

Despite stating the above, the authors go on to say that the mainstay of treatment for SIBO remains antibiotic treatment. They do, however, indicate that in many cases the relief is only temporary. Although many antibiotics have been used, the one most used is rifaximin.

Despite antibiotics continuing to be the treatment of choice for many mainstream doctors, it is important to note that since most bacteria live in biofilms, antibiotics may not be that useful. (More about biofilms later).

Another perspective to consider is that just killing off the causative bacteria is not the answer: we must deal with the predisposing factors. The Dukowicz, Lacy, and Levine paper does not adequately address the first two points mentioned above.

The natural approach to treating SIBO

- Treat the hypochlorhydria. This can be achieved by simple things such as ACV, betaine HCL or lemon juice before each meal.
- Treat the gall bladder. This can be done by stimulating bile flow. The use of a herbal cholagogue (herb to increase bile flow) can be useful, the simplest one is to drink regular cups of dandelion root tea (*Taraxicum officinale*), generally easily available from the supermarket. It is also helpful to supplement with two specific amino acids, taurine, and glycine. Both are needed for bile production. Ox bile supplements may also be helpful especially where there has been a cholecystectomy, or the previously mentioned treatments are not producing adequate results.
- Herbal antibiotics can be used, e.g., berberine, oils of oregano, cloves, and thyme. Chedid et al. (2014) demonstrated that these natural antibiotic herbal oils are as good as rifaximin without the side effects. The researchers also showed that in cases where rifaximin failed, the people responded to the herbal therapies better. We will see later that these herbs work better because they can break up the biofilms.
- Dietary changes. Avoid high roughage foods as mentioned earlier, and possibly the best change, at

least at the beginning of treatment, is to recommend a low FODMAP eating pattern.

- Probiotics should always be used, especially if conventional antibiotic treatment has been used sometime in the past. If antibiotics have been used patients may develop a secondary candida over-growth, so treatment with nystatin (conventional) or Pau d'Arco (non-conventional) may be used. Leventogiannis et al. (2019) demonstrated that probiotics have an effect in SIBO/IBS. Bustos Fernández, Man, and Lasa (2023) showed benefit with the use of the probiotic, Saccharomyces boulardii, which is a fungal probiotic.

- Acupuncture. Many studies have shown the benefit of acupuncture in gastrointestinal problems in general. Although the studies refer mainly to irritable bowel syndrome, remember that a large portion of these IBS could be SIBO. Another interesting study showed that acupuncture has a regulatory action on gastrointestinal function in general (Chan, Carr, & Mayberry, 1997; Takahashi, 2006; Schneider, Streitberger, & Joos, 2007; Li et al., 2015; Chao & Zhang, 2014).

- Treat the ICV. How do you know if there is an ICV problem? Generally, there is pain/discomfort when pushing on the right lower abdominal area, which, for the medically minded, is known as McBurney's point (named after American surgeon Charles

McBurney 1845–1913). An ICV that is stuck in the open position can cause SIBO with constant diarrhoea. Treatment consists of massaging the area or applying a cold pack to the area. An ICV that is stuck in the closed position which can lead to constipation can also be massaged. A magnesium supplement may help. There are many YouTube videos showing how to massage the area. Acupuncture may also help. Dietary changes as described above are also essential.

Biofilms

*"Some doctors make the same mistake for 20 years
and call it clinical experience."*
Voltaire (1694-1778)

Biofilm is another buzz word that has recently emerged. A good question to start with is, *"Where does the microbiome live?"* The answer is simple. In the gut of course, but where actually? Do they just float around in the gut? No. Although some do float freely, most exist in biofilms.

What is a biofilm? Brackman and Coenye (2015) defined a biofilm as *"microbial sessile communities characterised by cells that are attached to a substratum or interface or to each other, are embedded in a self-produced matrix of extracellular polymeric substances* (EPS) *and exhibit an altered phenotype compared to planktonic cells."*

Note: planktonic cells are free-floating bacteria.

Bacteria in a biofilm live attached to the walls of the gut, mouth, teeth, vagina, skin, nose, and sinuses, and in wounds anywhere and everywhere. And they act differently to their free-floating comrades. They are the same species, but they seem to switch on a completely different physiology.

They can also grow outside the body attached to surfaces, walls, pipes, etc. They are hard to eliminate. They may need to be physically removed, physically scrubbed clean. Just spraying antiseptics will not work.

Biofilms stop wounds from healing and infect burns. The scum on the teeth that forms cavities is a biofilm, they can form in the bladder, which leads to recurrent bladder infections, and are difficult to treat with antibiotics. They can stick to medical devices such as artificial heart valves, catheters, and joint replacements. They are hard to eradicate. A good example is the chronically infected tonsils where biofilms form and antibiotics do not work: the treatment may have to be a tonsillectomy.

Biofilms clump together for defensive purposes and communicate with each other using chemical messaging. Bacteria can sense other bacteria in the vicinity with these chemical messages called quorum sensing (QS). Just as in any meeting, a certain number of attendees is needed to form the quorum so that the meeting has legitimacy, so when the messages and therefore the number of bacteria, reach a critical mass, it is called a "quorum". Once the bacteria reach this critical mass, they flock together and form a biofilm, they can "talk"/communicate with each other and can even diversify. Some in the clump take on different roles than others, which means they can act like a multicellular organism. They do this for four main reasons:

- to protect themselves (defence),
- to colonize themselves in a nutrient-rich area,
- for utilization of cooperative benefits, and
- because biofilms are the default mode of growth.

This is really interesting. According to Jefferson (2004), the free bacteria that we see in the lab are an artefact. Although there are some free-floating bacteria around, bacteria normally exist in biofilms.

There is evidence that biofilms can be caused by antibiotic treatment. The bacteria naturally want to protect themselves, so biofilms are formed. Certainly, low dose antibiotics can do this, *"...subinhibitory concentrations (subMICs) of antibiotics have an important role in evolution of antibiotic resistance and induction on biofilm formation"* (Yuksel, Karatug, & Akcelik, 2018).

In another study, Kaplan (2011) found that *"...low dose antibiotics induce bacterial biofilm formation."*

Hoffman et al. (2005) reported that biofilm formation can be a specific defence mechanism to the presence of aminoglycoside antibiotics.

This can be a conundrum. Considering the above, how is it possible to treat infections when antibiotics may produce biofilms, which then make the bacteria causing the infection even more difficult to eradicate? It is important, that if antibiotics are used, then they must be full strength, and in high, or adequate, doses. Low doses may produce biofilms.

The bacteria in the biofilm are hard to eradicate. They are relatively resistant to antibiotics. Antibiotics deal with the free-floating bacteria quite well but not the biofilms. As above, the first reason is to protect themselves. Bacteria aren't stupid. They do not want to be killed off, so they form a biofilm to protect themselves. What is the best way to deal with the biofilms? Since antibiotics do not really work, they may need to be physically removed. Young, Morton, and Bartley (2010) showed that biofilms in chronic rhinosinusitis can be physically disrupted using ultrasound.

One innovative way is to target the chemical messaging system. This system allows one bacterium to sense when there is another nearby.

Blocking the messaging, then, is one way to stop biofilm formation. If this is done, one bacterium will *not* know if there is another one nearby because the message would not get through, so they would not form a quorum and develop into a biofilm. Here the idea of a quorum sensing inhibitor (QSI) or "anti-quorums" comes in. The interesting thing is that many of the traditional anti-bacterial herbs used for generations have anti-quorum or QSI properties. Some of these herbs are:

- garlic (Jakobsen et al., 2012)
- cranberry (LaPlante, Sarkisian, Woodmansee, Rowley, & Seeram, 2012)
- oregano (Lee, Kim, & Lee, 2017)
- curcumin (Vaughn et al., 2017)
- sage (Al-Bakri, Othman, & Afifi, 2010)
- berberine (Zhang et al., 2022)
- cloves (Khan, Zahin, Hasan, Husain, & Ahmad, 2009)
- tea tree oil (Kwieciński, Eick, & Wójcik, 2009)
- apple cider vinegar, external use in wounds (Bjarnsholt et al., 2015)
- colloidal silver (Goggin, Jardeleza, Wormald, & Vreugde, 2014)

Another substance that has been shown to break up biofilms is caprylic acid – a component of coconut oil. Rosenblatt et al. (2017) demonstrated that a combination of caprylic acid and polygalacturonic acid, also known as pectic acid (from ripe fruits, e.g., apples, pears) eradicated biofilms and inhibited the growth of planktonic organisms. Caprylic acid on its own was good but the combination of the two was much better. However, this was done in an *in vitro* experiment, i.e., in a petri dish, not in a living body.

Pandit et al. (2017) demonstrated that ascorbate/vitamin C can reduce and disrupt biofilms. Even low concentrations of vitamin C reduces the synthesis of the extracellular polymeric substances (EPS) and destabilizes bacterial biofilms. This can expose the bacteria and kill them by the oxidative action of vitamin C, or by other antimicrobial treatments. El-Mowafy, Shaaban, and Abd El Galil (2014) showed that sodium ascorbate has quorum sensing inhibition of Pseudomonas infection.

MTHFR, methylation and the gut

"There are no difficult cases, only difficult patients."
Zhou Jian Ling

The above words are often heard these days although they are not always understood. Like other words mentioned previously, methylation and associated words and concepts have become popular. What then, is methylation? And what does MTHFR stand for? There are many concepts involved including, genetics, biochemistry, and nutrition. Following is a simplified explanation of this complex concept, hopefully made easier to understand as I go beyond the science to show how it all fits together.

MTHFR (*Methyl TetraHydroFolate Reductase*) is just one enzyme that is essential in the final activation of folate. The only folate the body can use is in the form of methyl tetrahydrofolate (MTHF), no other forms of folate will do. The gene that encodes for this enzyme is the MTHFR gene. When the human genome project was

113

finalised, they found that many genes have variations (I call them variations, not mutations) called single nucleotide polymorphisms (SNP, often referred to as "snips"). This variation is where one amino acid is substituted for another. This one change can make a difference, especially if the change is in a critical position.

The bigger the protein, the less the SNP has an effect. This change may be enough to alter the shape the protein or enzyme folds into, and since function is related to shape, this alteration of just one amino acid in that one critical position is enough to alter function. This means that not everyone has the exact same gene. A protein is a string of amino acids. Imagine it like a string of pearls, and one of the pearls is a different shape; the pearls then do not sit correctly.

Note that this does not only occur with the MTHFR gene: every gene in your body can potentially have SNPs. The whole genome can be tested to see which genes have SNPs. There may be thousands. This whole process can get very complicated but then you can see which genes have SNPs and therefore work out where your metabolism can go wrong, and which nutrients are needed to supplement to get over this blockage. We must resist the idea that if we test only for the MTHFR gene, and SNPs are found, then we must automatically treat that one gene.

Many practitioners, especially early on, automatically prescribed methyl B12, and/or 5 methyltetrahydrofolate (MTHF) when they saw a MTHFR SNP. This is wrong because as I said earlier, there are thousands of SNPs in the body. They are generally in balance and this approach may lead to unfortunate outcomes.

Physiology and biochemistry teach that enzymes are needed to drive the various metabolisms. Nutritional medicine teaches that each enzyme has co-factors, e.g., zinc, or magnesium or vitamin B6. So, to help the reaction, we can supplement the co-factors to help the reaction along.

Nutritional medicine is applied biochemistry.

The next level of complexity is the "promotors" and "inhibitors". These are not necessarily directly involved in the reaction. Promotors include substances such as S-Adenosyl-Methionine (SAMe), so to promote the enzyme that needs SAMe, we can improve methylation or supplement SAMe. Other promotors include various amino acids and hormones such as cortisol, oestrogen, and progesterone.

Another example of a "promotor" is lipopolysaccharides (LPS) which are large molecules consisting of a lipid and a polysaccharide that are bacterial toxins. LPS are not good to have in the system (see section on leaky gut syndrome) as they can cause inflammation. LPS is a promotor for an enzyme that is activated by inflammation. LPS promotes an inhibiting reaction.

In some ways co-factors and activators are similar. In some cases, SAMe is a promotor but can also be an inhibitor and in some cases, it can be a co-factor. That is how important this substance is. The levels of SAMe can act in a positive or a negative feedback loop.

Inhibitors have a negative effect on the enzyme and may be environmental agents, such as toxins and chemicals, or heavy metals such as lead, mercury, cadmium, etc. In other situations, SAMe can also be an inhibitor. In certain situations, a high SAMe inhibits and a low SAMe promotes. From this we can see that we can help our enzymes by improving our nutrition and by cleaning up our environment.

Eating healthier, avoiding pollution, avoiding chemicals in the home such as cleaning products, removing mercury from our teeth and various other actions, all serve to improve our health.

Once we learn the biochemical pathways, we can supplement the co-factors to help the enzyme work optimally. We can improve our environment by reducing the enzyme inhibitors, therefore we do have some control over our biochemistry. Now, with the SNPs, it gets even more complicated because some SNPs make the enzyme work faster, and other SNPs can make the enzyme work slower. Co-factors can still be used.

Other options are:

- to supplement the end-product, which basically by-passes the (slow) enzyme block, or
- to give herbs or supplements that can slow down or speed up the variant enzyme.

This is good in the synthesis phase but not as good in the breaking down phase. For example, the co-factors for MTHFR are vitamins B2 and B3. This is my preferred starting point. However, we can supplement the end-product which is 5 methyl tetrahydrofolate (5 MTHF), but this must be done carefully and not necessarily as the first choice.

Another example is *catechol o methyltrasferase* (*COMT*), the enzyme involved in dopamine breakdown. There is a "fast *COMT*" and a "slow *COMT*"!

The "fast *COMT*" breaks down dopamine too quickly, therefore the levels of dopamine are low, which can lead to low motivation, addictions and depression. We must raise dopamine levels by slowing down the "fast COMT" with an herb such as rhodiola (*Rhodiola rosea)*, and we can also supplement tyrosine, the precursor of dopamine.

The "slow *COMT*" metabolises dopamine too slowly and leads to higher levels of dopamine, noradrenaline and adrenaline which can lead to anxiety, aggression, schizophrenia, impulsivity, violence etc. We need to lower dopamine by reducing tyrosine in the diet. Here a low protein diet may help, as well as improving methylation, and supplementing SAMe, magnesium and improving liver phase 2.

These variations are relatively common and having this variation does not necessarily produce disease. The following quote is paraphrased from one in Dr Andrew Rostenberg's book, *Your Genius Body*.

> Remember that the gene is your tendency not your destiny!

There are two common variants on the MTHFR gene, at positions 677 and 1298. These seem to be the critical areas. There may be more, but these are not tested because they do not seem to have any major effects. The numbers refer to the position of the change. A single variation at position 677 is referred to as being C667T heterozygote. Two variations at 677 is referred to as being homozygote.

Remember that you have two sets of genes: one from mum and one from dad. You can also have a single variation at 1298; heterozygote and two variations as homozygote. Another situation is the "compound heterozygote" where there is one variation at 677 and one at 1298. So, we can see that the MTHFR enzyme can have many variations, which leads to the enzyme not working optimally. Remember that this is just one gene, think of all the combinations and permutations if hundreds of other genes are considered. Although this gene is significant, it helps to look at the big picture, not just focus on one gene.

Methylation is the process of transferring a methyl group from a donor molecule to a gene, lipid, or protein. The body's major methyl donor is S-Adenyl-Methionine (SAMe), therefore the production of SAMe is a very important process. The methylation cycle works billions of times every second in every cell of our body. It is extremely important and is, in fact, fundamental to the effective working of each one of those cells.

Methylation is involved in:

- switching cellular function on and off,
- maintaining RNA and DNA and is therefore needed in cell replication. Human gut cell turnover is every four to five days. Methylation can protect DNA so is important in cancer,
- turning genes on and off. (Involved in epigenetics; epigenetics is the study of how the outside environment turns our genes on and off),
- turning enzymes on and off,
- turning neurotransmitters on and off,

- turning on tissue repair,
- turning off inflammation,
- turning the stress response on and off,
- protecting telomeres, therefore reducing the aging process,
- detoxifying chemicals by producing glutathione, the body's main detoxifier,
- producing energy because methylation is needed for ATP production and needed by the mitochondria,
- metabolising various proteins such as histamine.

The above list shows how important methylation is and why problems can present in many ways.

The folate cycle drives the SAMe production cycle, as well as serotonin/dopamine neurotransmitter production.

If the folate cycle is slow (because of a variant MTHFR enzyme) then the production of SAMe is reduced, and a low level, or slow production of SAMe affects methylation. A slow folate cycle can also affect the production of neurotransmitters leading to anxiety, depression, and other mental health issues.

Although things may not be as simple as this. There are SNPs that slow down methylation and there are SNPs that possibly can speed up methylation. The whole body can act like a "tug of war" scenario. Most healthy people have the situation where all the SNPs are balanced.

This affects the gut in many ways:

- SAMe is needed in the breakdown of serotonin and dopamine, not just in the brain but also the gut. Refer to the discussion about how the gut makes and uses these neurotransmitters.
- SAMe is needed to make new healthy gut cells because methylation is needed in DNA and RNA synthesis. The gut epithelial cells are constantly being turned over; they are replaced every four to five days. Poor replacement of the gut cells can lead to loss of epithelial integrity or barrier function (LGS, SIBO) or even to cancer (Sheaffer et al., 2014).
- SAMe is needed to breakdown histamine (histamine will be discussed later).

Note that stress inhibits methylation.

So, you can see that SIBO can influence methylation and methylation can affect the gut.

Methylation is also needed in gall bladder function. Part of methylation is the production of taurine which is essential in optimal bile function. It has been stated that the gall bladder is the most methylation sensitive organ in the body. If the gall bladder is not making bile, then this can lead to SIBO.

(https://www.beyondmthfr.com/mthfr-digestion-methylation-connection-gallbladder-function/ accessed 11 May 2023)

Leaky gut syndrome (LGS), which will be discuss in detail later, is also a factor in this context. Because methylation is needed for proper cell replication, especially in the gut, poor methylation can lead to a leaky gut. Toxins from bacteria notably LPS can damage gut cells and since gut cells are already not optimal with methylation issues, then LPS can enter the blood stream and cause varying issues such as inflammation, pain, brain fog, etc. LPS can also further impair methylation by affecting the enzyme *methionine adenosyl transferase* (MAT) which is the enzyme that converts methionine to SAMe; this is a vicious cycle.

So, if there is an MTHFR SNP problem, and/or a methylation problem, where do we start treatment? The answer is quite simple. We start with fixing up the gut. How do we do that? Read this book to find out! The strategies I discuss are all part of healing the gut.

Histamine

Most people would recognise the name and would immediately think of allergies when they hear it. You know that you need to take an <u>anti</u>histamine for your hay fever.

Histamine has many functions. It is a neurotransmitter in your central nervous system (CNS), is necessary for stomach acid release and is involved in your immune system. In the brain, histamine promotes wakefulness (note that older antihistamines can make you drowsy), controls feeding behaviour, motivation and goal directed behaviours. Abnormal histamine signalling can be related to PD and MS (Passani, Panula, & Lin, 2014).

In the stomach, a hormone called *gastrin* causes a release of histamine which stimulates the acid producing parietal cells in the stomach to release acid. The older anti-acid drugs such as cimetidine and ranitidine were histamine receptor 2 (H2) blockers.

The pH of the stomach is monitored, so when it becomes too low, i.e., too acidic, a hormone called *somatostatin* is released. This has a suppressing effect on the parietal cells as well as suppressing the release of gastrin and histamine. So too much histamine does not necessarily produce too much acid.

Histamine can cause an immediate inflammatory response (hence allergies), it is a red flag for the immune system. It is stored in the mast cells and basophils and is released when they are stimulated. Histamine causes blood vessels to dilate. This allows white cells to quickly get to the site of action. Further to this, histamine in the gut can increase permeability and therefore lead to a leaky gut syndrome. So, it is an essential component of your body. It is when there is too much histamine that a problem arises. A potential consequence of an excess of histamine is "histamine intolerance." When this occurs, a person may react abnormally to the histamine. This excess occurs either because it cannot be broken down, or there is too much in the diet.

The epidemic of heartburn is not, as some have posited, an effect of too much histamine, but is mostly a product of a high carbohydrate diet. A high fat/low carbohydrate diet reduced GORD (Pointer, Rickstrew, Slaughter, Vaezi, & Silver, 2016).

When there is histamine intolerance, you may develop symptoms such as:

- headache/migraine,
- difficulty falling off to sleep, easy arousal,
- hypertension,
- vertigo or dizziness,
- arrhythmia or accelerated heart rate,

- difficulty regulating body temperature,
- anxiety,
- nausea, vomiting,
- abdominal cramps,
- flushing,
- nasal congestion, sneezing, difficult breathing,
- abnormal menstrual cycle,
- hives,
- fatigue,
- tissue swelling.

High histamine levels can be caused by SIBO, LGS, *diamine oxidase* (DAO) deficiency, high histamine foods and by reduced methylation.

DAO is a gut enzyme that breaks histamine down before it is absorbed. DAO production can be stimulated by nutrients such as vitamin B6, magnesium and copper. A higher protein diet also helps, as well as olive oil. Oleic acid – mainly omega 9 - a major component of olive oil has been shown to dramatically increase DAO. Balancing the omega 3/omega 6 ratio can also help. The western diet has excessively high omega 6, so, reduce omega 6 (plant oils such as canola) and increase omega 3 (fish oil) fatty acids (Wollin, Wang, & Tso, 1998).

Causes of a low DAO

- gluten intolerance,
- LGS,
- SIBO,
- DAO blocking foods - alcohol, energy drinks, tea,
- inflammation - CrD, UC,
- medications -
  - NSAIDs - aspirin, ibuprofen,
  - antidepressants - cymbalta, effexor, prozac, zoloft,
  - histamine (H2) blockers - cimetidine, ranitidine,
  - antihistamines - zyrtec, polaramine, phenergan,
  - It is interesting to note here that antihistamines can lower DAO.
  - anti-arrhythmics - propranolol, metoprolol, cardizem and
  - immune modulators - humira, enbrel, plaquenil.

A low DAO means that histamine is not broken down in the gut, the histamine can therefore cause the leaky gut syndrome and more histamine can be absorbed into the body. In conjunction with this, if there is a high histamine diet, then a bad situation can be compounded (Maintz & Novak, 2007).

Histamine-rich foods

- fermented alcoholic beverages
- fermented foods – such as sauerkraut, Kimchi, vinegar, soy sauce, kefir, and yoghurt
- vinegar containing foods – such as pickles and olives
- cured meats – such as bacon, salami, luncheon meats, hot dogs
- soured foods – such as sour cream, sour milk, soured bread
- dried fruits – such as apricots, prunes, dates, figs, raisins
- most citrus fruits
- aged cheese
- nuts – such as walnuts, cashews, peanuts
- vegetables – specifically avocados, eggplant, spinach, and tomatoes
- smoked fish and certain species of fish, such as mackerel, tuna, anchovies and sardines

To complicate matters, histamines that are already in the body, are released by certain foods (histamine liberators) such as alcohol, bananas, chocolate, cow's milk, nuts, papaya, pineapple, shellfish, strawberries, tomatoes, wheat germ and many artificial preservatives and dyes. As you can see there is an overlap with high histamine foods.

Patients have told me that they are allergic to strawberries because they develop a rash. However, it could be that the strawberries are acting as a histamine liberator rather than the patient being allergic to the fruit.

Note that although some of the foods mentioned are healthy and have been advocated in this book, they may not be good for you if you have a methylation/MTHFR problem or a DAO deficiency.

Note that I advocate a "low histamine diet" and not a "no histamine diet".

"What is food to one, is to others bitter poison".
Lucretius (96 BC – 55 BC)

Histamine-free foods you can eat

- anything fresh; meat, poultry (frozen is OK)
- fresh caught fish
- eggs
- gluten free grains, rice, quinoa
- fresh fruits
- fresh vegetables except for tomatoes, spinach, avocado and eggplant
- dairy substitutes; coconut milk, rice milk, hemp milk
- cooking oils, olive, coconut
- leafy herbs
- herbal teas

Note that the low histamine diet avoids dairy and grains/gluten which has been a common theme all throughout this book.

As stated earlier, histamine is broken down in the gut by DAO but once it gets into the body, another enzyme, *histamine n methyltransferase* (HMT) is needed for metabolism. This is one of those enzymes that transfers a methyl group from SAMe to another molecule. For histamine to be inactivated, it needs to be methylated, (it then is no longer histamine) and for this,

SAMe is needed. Therefore, a well working methylation cycle and possibly a well-functioning MTHFR is needed. If there are allergies, such as asthma and hay fever, then consider the possibility of high histamine and/or methylation problems.

The histamine content of food increases because of microbial fermentation, hence fermented foods are high in histamine. What about the bacteria in our gut microbiota? There are gut bacteria that produce histamine such as *Lactobacillus* species – *L. bulgaricus, L. casei, L. lactis L. reuteri and L. delbrueckii,* and *Enterococus* species, *Klebsiella*, *Enterobacter* and *Citrobacter*. To maintain the balance there are histamine-degrading bacteria such as *Bifidobacteria* species, other *Lactobacillus* species especially *L. rhamnosus, L. salivarius and L. planetarium* (Puglin et al., 2017).

The name of the game is balance. This balance is broken down when there is dysbiosis and/or SIBO or other gut issues.

Diverticular disease (DD)

"The physician does not learn everything he must know and master at high colleges alone. From time to time he must consult old women, gypsies, magicians, wayfarers and all manner of peasant folk and random people, and learn from them, for these have more knowledge about such things than all the high colleges."
Paracelsus (1493? -1541)

DD is a condition where the inside lining of the colon herniates out through the weak areas between the circular fibres of the muscles of the large intestine forming pockets called diverticulae. They are more common in the sigmoid colon. The incidence is about 10% in the over 45 age group and increases to 65% in the over 70 age group.

The following are some terms that many confuse:

- Diverticular disease is the general term.

- Diverticulosis is where there are diverticulae present.
- Diverticulitis is where the diverticulae have become inflamed or infected.

This out-pocketing is thought to be due to increased pressure in the colon largely due to the low fibre western diet.

Only fifteen to twenty percent of those who have DD develop symptoms. Of these a quarter develop inflammation. Bleeding is very rare.

If the diverticulae become inflamed or infected then symptoms, such as pain, fever, a change in bowel habits, and blood or mucous in the stools, can develop. DD is conveniently divided into "uncomplicated" and "complicated".

Uncomplicated DD can be treated with simple measures at home, under appropriate medical supervision. Complicated DD, however, may cause bowel perforation, peritonitis, abscesses, bleeding, or fistulae, all of which needs hospital treatment and, in some cases, surgery.

What predisposes to DD?

Diet. Many studies show that a low fibre diet can predispose to DD. Studies in underdeveloped countries show that DD is virtually unknown and did not emerge until the introduction of a low fibre western diet (Korzenik, 2006).

The reason a high fibre diet is considered more effective in reducing the potential for DD is that if there is low bulk in the colon, the muscles must work harder to move the low bulk along thus increasing the pressure. A higher bulk is moved forward easier with less pressure.

There is some evidence that eating red meat may predispose to DD. Manousos et al. (1985) found a 50-fold difference in DD between those that frequently consume vegetables and rarely eat meat with those that rarely consume vegetables and frequently eat meat. So, the question is *"Is it the excess meat or the lack of vegetables?"*

Aldoori et al. (1994) supported the hypothesis that a diet low in total dietary fibre increases the incidence of symptomatic DD, although *"high intake of total fat or red meat and a diet low in total dietary fiber particularly augments the risk."*

So, again we ask the question – *"Is it the meat or a lack of vegetables?"*

As mentioned above, a lack of fibre/vegetables does greatly increase the risk of DD.

As for red meat, Cao et al. (2018) studied meat intake and DD, although this study was an observational study based on a recall questionnaire which always has bias issues and thus cannot produce a firm conclusion about cause and effect. They found that if poultry or fish was substituted for one serving a day there was a 20% reduction of risk. The study also noted that those who ate higher quantities of red meat also tended to use NSAIDs more, use more painkillers, smoked more, were less likely to exercise and had a lower fibre intake. Those that ate more poultry and fish were more likely to exercise more and to smoke less. Smoking, exercise and NSAID intake are other factors that can predispose to DD. So, the consumption of red meat must not be taken out of context with fibre and other factors. However, in this study, after taking all the influential factors into account, the researchers still concluded that it was the total red meat intake that was significant. They found that the risk peaked at six servings of red meat a week.

Obesity. Strate, Liu, Aldoori, Syngal, and Giovannucci (2009) showed that obesity increases risks of diverticulitis and diverticular bleeding.

Exercise. Williams (2009) showed that exercise reduces the incidence of DD. Strate, Liu, Aldoori, and Giovannucci (2009) demonstrated that exercise also decreases the incidence of diverticular complications.

Use of aspirin and NSAIDs. There is increased risk of diverticulitis and bleeding with the use of these medications (Strate, Liu, Huang, Giovannucci, & Chan, 2011).

Smoking. Smoking is found not only to predispose to DD, but smokers are more likely to develop complications and the complications proceed more rapidly (Aune et al., 2017; Turunen et al., 2010).

Dr Peter Baratosy MBBS FACNEM

DD prevention

We have become a nation of obese, low vegetable eating, non-exercising people who take lots of pain killers and NSAIDs. Thankfully smoking rates have decreased. Obviously, looking at the above factors, the best way to prevent DD is to eat more fibre, more fruits, vegetables, and salads. It is preferable to eat less red meat. However, you can still eat meat but vary the types of meat to include fish, and chicken, as well as beef, lamb, and other meats. Avoid obesity, exercise more, don't smoke and don't take aspirin and/or NSAIDs unnecessarily.

Treatment of DD

The sudden onset of abdominal pain can be quite frightening especially for the first time. A diagnosis must be made, so in this situation a visit to the doctor or to the hospital is a must. On first presentation, a CT scan can be quite useful partly to make a definite diagnosis but also to assess whether it is an uncomplicated or a complicated situation. Obviously if this is not your first attack, then you may be able to judge, based on your previous experience, the severity, although you may still want to go to the hospital. Obviously, prevention is better than cure, so follow the advice as above.

Uncomplicated DD can be treated conservatively. Initially, during an acute attack, a temporary low fibre diet may be useful. A soft diet of bone broth, vitamised veggies and other easily digested foods is the best as it is necessary to "give the gut a rest". Other measures, which have been discussed elsewhere in the book may also be initiated. These include soothing and healing the gut with SEB or aloe vera, glutamine, probiotics, anti-inflammatory herbs such as curcumin, anti-infective herbs such as berberine and garlic, as well as omega 3 fatty acids. Pain relief can be achieved with PEA or MC. Standard conventional analgesics can also be used. Also, it is helpful to increase exercise as tolerated.

One of the probiotics found useful in DD is EcN which Fric and Zavoral discussed in 2003. Their study results showed that the probiotic *"significantly prolonged the remission period and improved the abdominal syndrome in uncomplicated diverticular disease."*

Andersen et al. (2012) found that there is no evidence for the routine use of antibiotics in uncomplicated cases, although they may be used in selected cases depending on the overall condition.

Complicated DD probably will need hospital admission, with intensive treatment, antibiotics, surgery, and possibly other invasive procedures. This is not within the scope of this book.

Dysbiosis

"There is a pill for every ill and a bill for every pill."
Unknown

"There is a pill for every ill and an ill for every pill."
Prof. Anton Jayasuriya

It is well known that our colon is full of bacteria. We, therefore, to be well, must be in balance with these bacteria. When we are out of balance, we become sick. Isn't this what is happening in our society? So many are sick with digestive and abdominal problems.

Dr Peter Baratosy MBBS FACNEM

The gut microbiome

What is the microbiome? This is another word that has come into common use in the past decade. The microbiome is the sum total of trillions of microorganisms that live in the gut. The gut is only one niche of the whole human microbiota. Not only do microorganisms live in the gut, but they are also on our skin, in the mouth, the vagina, in fact, almost everywhere. A recent report from the ABC (ABC News 3 June 2018) has shown that a microbiome even exists in the bladder.

The gut as the second brain

This is a good time to introduce the topic of the gut-brain connection. The gut is a very complex organ, it is not just a tube from the mouth to the anus. Recent findings (Spencer et al., 2018) have made it even more complicated. Other than the trillions of gut microorganisms that reside in the gut there is also a complex array of over 100 million nerve cells or neurons. There are even more nerve cells in the gut than in the spinal cord (Sonnenburg & Sonnenburg, 2015).

The second brain is the gut. All these nerves are not just for local control, as there is a two-way connection to and from the "main" brain. The enteric nervous system (ENS) not only controls the gut but can signal and influence the "main" brain, including how it processes thoughts and emotions. For many years, we have connected the brain with the gut without really thinking about it. This is shown through common phrases that have entered our language. We have a "gut feeling", we "hate your guts" "you are a pain in the arse", then we get "butterflies in the stomach" when nervous, and we may "poop our pants" when scared. We get abdominal discomfort and bloating when anxious. There is a close relationship between the adrenal glands and the gut, and our gut is very responsive to our emotions, especially anxiety and stress. When we are stressed, the initial reaction is the "flight or fight" response. The body shunts blood to the muscles so that we can run faster or fight harder. As digestion is not a priority when running or fighting, blood supply is diverted from the gut and therefore the gut suffers.

The human body has not developed a chronic stress mechanism, it just uses the acute "fight or flight" reaction repeatedly.

The gut connects to the brain to influence emotions and the brain also connects to the gut to influence its function.

To keep our gut and brain happy we must eat well. Part of the ENS is the interaction between the nerve cells and the gut bacteria, so it is essential to have a good gut microbiome. We can take probiotic supplements but eating foods like yoghurt, kefir, kombucha, sauerkraut, kimchi, etc. will also improve our microbiome and as an extension, our brain.

Supplementing *Acidophilus, or Bifidobacterium* is good, but there may be a better way. Special strains have been shown to have different effects on the body, so it is a good idea to choose special probiotic strains or species for specific conditions (Ciorba, 2012).

The gut not only has the ENS, the two-way connection of the gut to the brain, but the two parts of the autonomic nervous system (ANS) are also involved.

There is the parasympathetic connection via the Vagus nerve and the sympathetic connection via the prevertebral ganglia. The gut can also make neurotransmitters, such as serotonin, dopamine, GABA, and many others. The role of serotonin in the gut is probably the most studied.

You may think that these neurotransmitters are made only by the brain. No. The gut makes more. For example, about 90% of the serotonin in the body is made by the gut. Any change in gut serotonin can lead to a wide variety of conditions ranging from the obvious irritable bowel syndrome to cardiovascular disease and osteoporosis. Yano et al. (2015) showed that certain spore producing bacteria, about twenty species in the microbiome, are important to production of serotonin in the gut. Without these specific bacteria, the production of serotonin is low. The serotonin produced by the gut has local effects as well as affecting the "main" brain indirectly. Serotonin produced in the gut affects:

- bowel motility,
- how much fluid, such as mucous, is produced by the gut, and
- how sensitive your gut is to pain or fullness after eating.

Some of the sensors send messages to the brain to produce a reflex nausea, bloating or pain, while locally it makes changes in sensitivity to pressure or pain (Sikander, Rana, & Prasad, 2009).

As in the brain, the gut not only makes serotonin but at least thirty other neurotransmitters. No doubt that is why it is called the second brain.

Selective serotonin reuptake inhibitors (SSRIs), which act to raise serotonin levels in the brain are used very commonly to treat depression. The downside is that there are many side effects to these drugs with a significant number related to the gut (Wang et al., 2022). Despite the benefits of increasing the availability of serotonin in the brain, SSRIs can also affect the microbiome. Sjöstedt, Enander, and Isung (2021) noted that *"They (i.e., SSRIs) also exhibit antimicrobial properties that comes with the potential of disrupting microbial hemostasis."*

The serotonin made in the gut is the same molecule that is made in the brain, but serotonin cannot cross the blood brain barrier (BBB). The local action of serotonin in the gut does affect the main brain and the effect of serotonin in the brain can influence the gut, although this seems to be an indirect effect largely mediated by the Vagus nerve and the prevertebral ganglia.

The gut can work independent to the brain. In the past, one of the surgical procedures performed for stomach ulcers was a vagotomy, the cutting of the Vagus nerve, and people did survive afterwards. Unfortunately, many were left with various gut problems caused by the loss of the gut brain connection (Liu & Forsythe, 2021).

Serotonin is found in some foods, such as walnuts, pineapples, bananas, kiwi fruit and tomatoes, so including these foods in the diet may be beneficial. However, although the serotonin in these foods cannot pass through the BBB, the building block of serotonin, the amino acid tryptophan, can.

Foods high in tryptophan are turkey, bananas, milk, yogurt, eggs, meat, nuts, beans, fish, and a variety of cheeses including Swiss and Cheddar.

However, the overall amount of tryptophan in food is quite low, so it can be difficult to obtain adequate amounts through food intake. Of all the amino acids, tryptophan, accounts for only about 1% and the absorption through the BBB is low due to competition with other amino acids. Carbohydrates are needed to help get tryptophan into brain. They stimulate insulin which pushes many amino acids into peripheral cells, which then leaves tryptophan an easier passage into the brain through the BBB. Once tryptophan enters the brain, carbohydrates remain the main stimulant for production of serotonin. The need for carbohydrates for serotonin production may explain why depressed people eat more carbs and why junk foods are so popular.

Carbohydrates are called "feel good foods" and this makes sense since they help to raise serotonin in the brain. It works in reverse as well. People on low carb diets become depressed due to low levels of serotonin. It is interesting that this effect seems to be stronger in women than men. So, the inclusion of low GI (glycaemic index) carbs in your diet is important.

We should consider this system not only as the brain-gut system but as the brain-gut-microbiome system. It is a two-way street mostly mediated via the Vagus nerve. The whole system is very complicated, but the focus for the next discussion will be on how the brain affects the gut and the microbiome, and how the microbiome affects the gut and the brain.

So basically, your gut can influence your mood. This was shown in a study looking at children's temperaments and associating it with their gut microbiome. Christian et al. (2015) compared children with "good" and "bad" temperaments and found significant differences in levels of various gut bacteria such as *Dialister*, *Rikenellaceae*, *Ruminococcaceae* and *Parabacteroides.*

Experiments with germ-free mice (mice with a germ-free gut) or germ-free rats, where microbiota from normal and diseased mice and/or humans are transplanted, show interesting results. This is colloquially known as "trans-poo-sition". Transferring the microbiota from a depressed human to a germ-free rat reproduces depression in a rat. My question is, how can you tell if a rat is depressed? Rats love sugar water and they cannot get enough of it but when they were given the microbiome of a depressed person, they no longer cared about the sugar water.

Cryan and Dinan (2012) demonstrated the concept of the microbiota-gut-brain, where the microbial composition of the gut can influence:

- immune activation,

- Vagus nerve signalling,

- alterations in tryptophan metabolism,

- production of specific microbial neuroactive metabolites, and

- alteration of bacterial wall sugars, which allows alteration in communication between the bacteria and the gut wall.

Transfer the microbiome and you transfer the behaviour or the disease.

Sampson et al. (2016) showed that PD in mice can be related to the microbiome. This study showed that transplanting the microbiota from humans with PD can produce Parkinson's-like symptoms in susceptible mice much worse than if the microbiota from healthy humans was transplanted. This doesn't happen only in mice. When PD patients are compared with non-PD patients, there is a great difference in the microbiome.

In PD patients there is a 77.6% reduction of *Prevotellaceae species.* Scheperjans et al. (2015) found another species, *Enterobacteriaceae,* appears to be linked to the severity of PD symptoms, especially postural instability and gait difficulty. The higher the levels, the worse the symptoms.

Villumsen, Aznar, Pakkenberg, Jess, and Brudek (2019) showed a strong correlation between IBD and PD, as well as multiple system atrophy (MSA). In theory, you can treat PD just by treating the gut. This gut/brain connection is probably mediated via the Vagus nerve.

A study by Liu et al. (2017) resulted in some evidence that a truncal vagotomy has a potential protective effect against PD while a selective vagotomy does not.

Changes to the microbiome have also been linked to diseases such as:

- allergy (Lynch & Boushey, 2016),

- obesity (Maruvada, Leone, Kaplan, & Chang, 2017),

- Alzheimer's disease (Jiang, Li, Huang, Liu, & Zhao, 2017),

- MS (Kirby & Ochoa-Repáraz, 2018). A progressive form of MS was shown to stabilise after a faecal transplant (Makkawi, Camara-Lemarroy, & Metz, 2018),

- IBD (Lane, Zisman, & Suskind, 2017), and

- autism (Luna, Savidge, & William, 2016; Mulle, Sharp, & Cubells, 2013).

As an extension of this idea, autism has been shown to respond to antibiotic treatment. This may not be an ideal form of long-term treatment but does strengthen the relationship of gut flora with autism (Sandler et al., 2000; Rodakis, 2015).

GI problems are a common comorbidity in autism. Li, Han, Dy, and Hagerman (2017) and Pulikkan, Mazumder, and Grace (2019) demonstrated a difference in the microbiome in children with autism, in particular a reduced number of *Bifidobacteria* and increased *Clostridium* spp, *Desulfovibrio* spp., *Sutterella* spp. and/or *Veillonellaceae*.

There are also changes to gut permeability with LGS noted by D'Eufemia et al. as far back as 1996.

Studies on the use of probiotics, prebiotics and dietary changes so far have shown conflicting results, although many parents are quite adamant that a gluten free and a dairy free diet have helped their autistic children.

In the above discussion evidence of the two-way communication, brain-gut and gut-brain can be seen.

What about faecal (poo) transplants? Kang et al. (2019), showed long term improvement in autism spectrum disorders after a poo transplant.

In humans, the gut microbiota is established by two years after birth and can be quite stable in a continuing healthy gut (see section on biofilms), but modern life is not good for our gut microorganisms. The microbiome starts at birth with a mouthful of vaginal bacteria as the baby passes through the birth canal. Jiménez et al. (2005) and Jiménez et al. (2008) demonstrated that there may be some gut microbial population occurring even before birth.

Willis et al. (2019) showed a fungal colonisation of the newborn gut.

The placenta may also have its own microbiome although this idea has been argued back and forth with some claiming the microbes found are due to contamination. At present we really do not know for sure. Aagaard et al. (2014) argue that there is a placental microbiome, while de Goffau et al. (2019) maintain that there is not a placental microbiome.

When considering the above, it is evident that if the baby is born by Caesarean section, they are already behind in the microbiome department. A good plan is to supplement Caesarean babies with a probiotic containing *Lactobacillus infantum*.

There is another option for mothers with a planned Caesarean section. Provide her with a container of sterile water and instruct her to insert a tampon into the vagina for half to one hour prior to the planned surgery. Then remove the tampon and place into the sterile water container. This technique is known as vaginal microbiota transfer (VMT) or vaginal seeding. It is important that this technique should only be done if the mother is known not to have any infectious diseases such as group B streptococcus, chlamydia, gonorrhoea, herpes, etc., which may then infect the baby.

After the baby is born, sterile cotton wool or gauze is used to wipe the water all over the baby. Zhou et al. (2023) proved that the babies that underwent this procedure had a more mature microbiota that was comparable to vaginally born babies, while the placebo group did not. The study also confirmed that the swabbed-on bacteria from the maternal vaginal fluid successfully reached and colonised the gut. The researchers then evaluated the babies at three months and six months and found that the babies scored significantly higher in neurodevelopment compared to the placebo babies (Caesarean babies that were exposed to sterile water only). These scores were comparable to vaginal born babies.

Kolokotroni et al. (2012) demonstrated that babies born with a Caesarean section have a poorer immunity and a higher incidence of allergies and asthma. This is more pronounced if there is a family history of atopy.

Some babies are cared for in neonatal intensive care, hopefully for good reason. Without the benefit of good maternal bacteria, these babies are more vulnerable to being colonised by other bacteria and various hospital microbes. Gut and immune maturation start at birth. Another concern is that too many children are given courses of antibiotics. Of course, in life and death infection situations, some may be essential. However, courses of antibiotics are sometimes given for trivial reasons. Antibiotics are not good for our gut bacteria.

Although the discussion has primarily focused on bacteria and the gut, the microbiome consists of much more than bacteria. Fungi, nematodes (worms), protists, archaea, and viruses are also important for a healthy microbiome, although little is known about the role of these organisms.

Back to the microbiome.

Most of the microorganisms live in the large intestine, many in biofilms. The stomach and small intestines are virtually devoid of any organisms.

In the colon there are an estimated 300 to 1000 different species, however 99% of the bacteria are comprised of only 30-40 different species. Over 90% of the bacteria are anaerobes. There are more bacteria genes in total than the human genome.

The microbiome can be divided into three categories:

Core: which accounts for about 60-70% of the species. This is the most stable in adulthood and is largely formed by geography, early life environment, genetics, etc. This pattern of species is so stable it can almost be considered as a fingerprint.

Variable: this accounts for 20-25% of species. This can vary with diet, seasons, medication, travel, and other health factors. This category is the one most affected by antibiotics, and possibly can recover, but slowly.

Transient: accounts for 5-15% of species. This is formed by microbes in the food, air, water, and this is the category that is influenced by probiotics.

Once established, the core microbiome is relatively stable; however, changes may occur related to lifestyle, diet, and age, although there are variations with individuals. This is why this subject can be so complicated.

Diet can have a significant effect on the microbiome. A bad diet can change the microbiome to become detrimental to one's health. Conversely a good diet can improve the microbiome to be beneficial to health. The most important factor seems to be adequate fibre. So, what is a healthy diet for your microbiome?

Singh et al. (2017) suggested that the Mediterranean diet is possibly the best. The researchers define the Mediterranean diet as being *"distinguished by a beneficial fatty acid profile that is rich in both monounsaturated and polyunsaturated fatty acids, high levels of polyphenols and other antioxidants, high intake of fiber and other low glycemic carbohydrates, and relatively greater vegetable than animal protein intake. Specifically, olive oil, assorted fruits, vegetables, cereals, legumes, and nuts; moderate consumption of fish, poultry, and red wine; and a lower intake of dairy products, red meat, processed meat and sweets..."*

There are four dominant phyla in the human gut: *Firmicutes, Bacteroidetes, Actinobacteria* and

Proteobacteria.

Fungal species have also been found including *Candida, Saccharomyces, Aspergillus, Penicillium, Rhodotorula, Trametes, Pleospora, Sclerotinia, Bullera and Galactomyces.*

The common species in the colon, in reverse order of frequency, are: Bacteroides fragilis, Bacteroides melaninogenicus, Bacteroides oralis, Enterococcus faecalis, Escherichia coli, Enterobacter species, Klebsiella species, Bifidobacterium bifidum, Staphylococcus aureus, Lactobacillus sp, Clostridium perfringens, Proteus mirabilis, Clostridium tetani, Pseudomonas aeruginosa.

If you have purchased a bottle of probiotics, you may find that hardly any of the bacteria on the above list are in the capsules. This is because it is not necessary to supplement all the above-mentioned bacteria. Probiotics do not replace the microbiome.

Probiotics, especially Lactobacillus rhamnosus GG and Saccharomyces boulardii, have been shown to restore the core bacteria (Korpela et al., 2016; Bajaj et al., 2014; Moré & Swidsinski, 2015).

It may come as a shock to the reader that most Lactobacillus species are not true intestinal inhabitants, they largely belong to the transient category (Walter, 2008).

Taking probiotics does not replace the microbiome but helps the gut improve its microbiota.

Another way to improve the microbiota is to supplement all the good bacteria. This is where the concept of the faecal microbiota transplant (FMT), otherwise known as the "poo transplant," developed. In some ways it makes sense. Clear out the colon of all organisms and "transplant" in the microbiome of a healthy person. Sounds simple in theory but not so in practice. Firstly, you need to clear the gut with powerful antibiotics, then you need healthy volunteers to act as donors.

There are alternatives, some people have done a "homemade" poo transplant. One woman used her husband's poo and administered it to herself via an enema. She made a good recovery from her *C. diff* infection. Nothing had helped prior. (BBC News 27 May 2014)

Note: Do not try this at home. It is not a recommendation: it is for information only.

However, Silverman, Davis, and Pillai (2010) discussed "self-administered faecal transplantation" using a low volume enema, for *Clostridium difficile (C. diff)* infection. The study of only 7 patients was small, but there was 100% success with a 14 month follow up. This method is certainly more inexpensive than the thousands of dollars you pay for a hospital poo transplant.

It is important for any transplant that the donor be healthy. As discussed earlier, conditions such as obesity, allergies, PD, Alzheimer's disease, and autism have a relationship to the gut microbiome. You do not want to get rid of one condition to then be burdened by another. The above papers reported on the use of the home-made poo transplant for *C. diff* infections. There is no reason this cannot be tried for other conditions such as PD, MS, autism, IBS, etc., as faecal transplant research, although still in early stages, has resulted in successful outcomes for these diseases.

Researchers are also now experimenting with freeze dried poo "crapsules" that you swallow like a probiotic. The poo comes from healthy donors. The protocol does not need antibiotics to kill off the existing microbiome before swallowing the "crapsules". Stalet et al. (2017) have shown this form of treatment to be superior to antibiotics in treatment of *Clostridium difficile (C.diff)* gut infection.

According to an article by Houser (2023), the FDA has already approved a pill made from human faecal matter to treat gut infections, notably *C. diff*. This treatment may potentially be effective for many other diseases.

(https://www.freethink.com/health/fecal-transplant-pill accessed 13 May 2023)

The relationship between us and our microbiome is not only a non-harmful coexistence but is also a mutual beneficial symbiotic relationship. The fibre in our diet feeds the microbiome and they, in return, do things for us. We must be in harmony with these bacteria, in other words, there must be a synergetic relationship between these bacteria and us. The bacteria of the microbiome are not the common or garden type, rather they are special bacteria, so-called "friendly" bacteria. From a simplistic point of view, the "friendly" bacteria balance out any "unfriendly" bacteria.

The bowel is full of bacteria weighing from 1.8-3 Kgs (4-7 pounds). When the bacteria are normal and in balance, they perform essential functions:

- They produce folate and vitamin B12. However, the B12 made in the colon cannot be absorbed because B12 can only be absorbed from the terminal ilium.
- They produce short chained fatty acids (SCFA), such as butyric acid from vegetable fibre. This nourishes the lining of the colon and may even reduce development of colon cancer.
- They inhibit harmful bacteria.
- They are important in destroying toxins.

The bowel is an eco-system and any deviation from this finely tuned balance will cause problems.

Then there are "bad" microorganisms. The colon can be infected with pathogenic organisms which can cause complications:

- bacteria such as Vibrio cholerae, Salmonella, Shigella, Clostridium difficile, Campylobacter, Yersinia, Klebsiella, Proteus and Citrobacter,
- parasites such as Entamoeba histolytica, Giardia lamblia, Dientamoeba fragilis, Blastocystis hominis, and
- yeasts such as Candida albicans. Candida is only a problem when the numbers are high, and the normal microbiome does contain some Candida.

For years many parents have been fanatically buying anti-worm tablets from the local pharmacy because the children have an itchy backside, or vague abdominal pains, or there is a case of worms in the school, or the pet dog has worms as diagnosed by the vet. People have been almost obsessed with killing off worms in the gut; however, worms in the gut can be part of the normal healthy microbiome. Worm eggs have been found in coprolites (fossilised poo) and in a Peruvian mummy from 900 BC. Worms were also found in the famed ice mummy, preserved in ice for 5,300 years, found at the Italian–Austrian border in 1991. The researchers named him Ötzi. Named thus due to the fact he was found in the Ötztal Alps.

So, are worms part of the normal microbiome?

Or are they always pathological?

Indian children are underweight, many have intestinal worms and 2-3% die between ages 1-6. Awasthi et al. (2013) studied one million children living in North India. The children were randomly divided into four groups and given either:

- vitamin A 200,000 IU capsule,
- albendazole 400 mgs capsule (anti worm drug),
- both,
- or neither, every 6 months for 5 years.

The results were interesting. The albendazole did reduce the incidence of worms but the treatment made no difference to the health or the death rate of the children.

Some researchers suggest that worms can be part of the normal microbiome. Ruyssers et al. (2008) showed that using worms can treat intestinal inflammation. Summers, Elliott, Urban, Thompson, and Weinstock (2005) demonstrated the benefits of using worms, specifically whipworm (Trichuris suis), in CrD. In the same year, the same group of researchers showed that the worms can also be used in treating UC (Summers, Elliott, Urban, Thompson, & Weinstock, 2005).

In the chapter on IBD, how worms have been used to treat IBD will be discussed.

Modern life is not good for our bacteria. Antibiotics are given indiscriminately for trivial conditions. Antibiotics are fed to animals and the residues are in the food we eat. These antibiotics kill off the good as well as the bad and upset this finely tuned balance. It is well known that after a course of antibiotics, many are not well, and they have various digestive problems. Many patients can think back and put the start of their troubles to a course of antibiotics, sometimes even years before.

Some cases may be temporary but in many cases the problem can be prolonged.

After any course of antibiotics, the "friendly" bacteria must be replaced. Naturopaths, other natural therapists, and integrative doctors have been advising people for years to take some form of friendly bacteria after a course of antibiotics, either in the form of yoghurt or as a probiotic supplement. This advice is now becoming mainstream.

Any dysregulation of this symbiotic balance between the person and their microbiome can lead to inflammatory and auto immune conditions.

Dysbiosis can be subdivided into four subcategories:

- **Putrefaction dysbiosis.** This is when the digestion of food is compromised. The food sits in our GI tract and literally rots. This causes symptoms of bloating, discomfort, indigestion, and smelly flatus.
- **Fermentation dysbiosis.** This is when the diet is high in sugars and carbohydrates. Instead of the food rotting the carbohydrates ferment, producing bloating, diarrhoea, and gas.
- **Deficiency dysbiosis.** This is due to deficiency of the "good" bacteria such as the lactobacilli. This is a very common occurrence today as it is caused by antibiotics as well as a low fibre diet.
- **Sensitisation dysbiosis.** This occurs when "bad" bacteria in the colon produce toxins, and the body recognises them as foreign. The leaky gut absorbs these toxins, and the body reacts to them. The concept of molecular mimicry and auto-immune diseases arose from the above premise and will be discussed further in the sections on leaky gut syndrome and molecular mimicry.

Candidiasis

Candidiasis is a specific form of dysbiosis.

Candidiasis generally refers to a condition which is thought to be caused by an over-growth of the yeast, *Candida albicans*, in the bowels. Some Candida does exist in the normal microbiome. Others think that there may be a hypersensitivity to the Candida.

Not everybody believes this. Many of the symptoms of "candidiasis" are so vague and general that it could be related to many other conditions. Mainstream medicine does not accept this concept.

On the other hand, the problems produced by poor digestion and lack of acid are enough to explain many of the symptoms patients describe, and the Candida overgrowth may be just a secondary overgrowth phenomenon.

However, there are some people with a set of symptoms that we can attribute to Candida overgrowth. If they follow a regime specifically designed to eliminate Candida, they do improve.

This may not be considered definite proof but for practical purposes, it is very convincing.

Symptoms of candidiasis include abdominal

bloating and gurgling, flatulence, especially odorous, itchy anus, and more systemic symptoms such as headache, fuzzy thinking, "foggy brain" and general fatigue. As mentioned earlier, these symptoms are not very specific. If everyone has some Candida in their bowel, and everyone does, why is it that one person may have problems, and another does not?

My opinion is that there is a syndrome, and it is related to Candida. Below, I outline the many reasons for why I believe there is such a syndrome.

If we assume that it exists, and we treat patients along the lines of Candida elimination and they get better, then it must mean that Candida has a role somewhere.

The treatment for candidiasis has much in common with overall treatment of digestive problems.

There is an eating plan designed to reduce, or even eliminate, sugars and carbohydrates from the diet. The theory is that since Candida is a yeast, it needs sugar to grow, so it must be starved.

One thing that most people should be aware of is that sugars and simple carbohydrates are not a healthy food to eat.

By eliminating sugars and many carbohydrates, the glycaemic load is reduced (carbohydrates are quickly metabolised to sugar). This treatment promotes health. Many ask if people get better because they are doing these healthy things, or because these healthy things kill off or starve Candida.

The answer is not simple, and the point can be debatable.

There is one detail, however, that makes me believe candidiasis exists and that is the positive effect seen with the use a specific anti-candida medication: *nystatin.*

Nystatin

Nystatin is a conventional medicine and is an antifungal antibiotic. It is active against yeasts and yeast-like fungi such as Candida. The mode of action of this antibiotic is thought to be due to its ability to bind sterols in the cell membranes, which increases the cell membrane permeability and causes intracellular components to leak out. Nystatin has no activity against bacteria.

Nystatin is virtually not absorbed from the gastro-intestinal tract (there are no detectable blood levels after standard dosing) and therefore has no systemic effects, i.e., it acts locally in the gut. Basically, it goes in one end, does its job in the gut, and then comes out the other end.

Although it is virtually not absorbed, there are very rare cases of hypersensitivity where the minuscule amount absorbed could cause allergic reactions. Excluding these very rare situations, nystatin is a very safe medication.

I prefer to use capsules and not tablets, as they are dispersed more easily and quickly and therefore have a much better action. The length of treatment depends on clinical response and can range from two weeks to indefinitely.

Side effects are minimal. Except the rare case of hypersensitivity, the most common side effects are gastro-intestinal distress, such as diarrhoea, nausea, and abdominal discomfort, although this is mainly when extra-large doses are used.

Some patients develop symptoms not related to the GI system and these are usually an aggravation of their symptoms of candidiasis. This is thought to be due to a Candida "die off." That is, as large numbers of Candida are killed, there is a massive release of toxins and proteins from the dying Candida, which are absorbed from the GI tract. The body reacts to these toxins and proteins in what is a form of Jarisch-Herxheimer reaction. Jarisch-Herxheimer reaction describes the release of endotoxins when many organisms are killed by antibiotics. This generally occurs with the treatment of syphilis but can also occur with other infections. Symptoms include fever, chills, headache, and myalgia.

Such a reaction can cause much discomfort and fortunately, or unfortunately, this is a sign of a successful treatment. Activated charcoal tablets, freely available from the local pharmacy can help to alleviate some of these symptoms.

People with symptoms of candidiasis do get better when nystatin is used. Why would using a specific anti-Candida medication work if the cause of the problem was not Candida?

Even if Candida is only a secondary problem, it still must be eliminated.

As already mentioned, many people can trace the onset of their problem to a course of antibiotics. It is well known that antibiotics kill bacteria, not just the harmful ones, but also the friendly ones. Many women suffer a bout of vaginal thrush after antibiotics. When the good bacteria are killed off along with the bad, Candida remains and overgrows because there is nothing to stop it. In the normal situation, the good bacteria keep Candida in check.

Santelmann, Laerum, Roennevig, and Fagertun (2001) tested nystatin with placebo in a group of "polysymptomatic" patients. This was a randomised, double blind, placebo-controlled trial and the conclusion was that *"Nystatin is superior to placebo in reducing localised and systemic symptoms in individuals with presumed fungus hypersensitivity as selected by a 7-item questionnaire. This superiority is probably enhanced even further by a sugar-and-yeast-free diet."*

See appendix 2 to view the 7-item questionnaire mentioned in the above paper.

Helicobacter pylori (HP)

Helicobacter pylori (previously known as Campylobacter pylori) can also be regarded as a form of dysbiosis, although there is evidence that perhaps it may be a normal commensal.

Two Australian researchers, Dr Barry Marshall and Dr Robin Warren, won the Nobel Prize in 2005 for their discovery that the bacterium Helicobacter pylori (HP) "caused" peptic ulcers and that antibiotics can be used to "treat" and "cure" ulcers.

My congratulations to them both.

The doctors were on the right track; however, I don't believe their research went quite far enough. Of course, antibiotics can be used to kill off bacteria. Doctors prescribe antibiotics all the time to treat tonsillitis, ear infections, SIBO or any other infection BUT the questions that should be asked are:

"Why does the body allow the bacteria to cause a problem?"

"Why is it that not everyone who has HP gets ulcers?"

A large percentage, estimates up to 50% of the population has been shown to have HP. The prevalence varies widely with geographic area, age, race, ethnicity, and social economic status. Studies have shown that HP has been living with humanity for a very long time. The first humans who migrated out of Africa carried HP with them. Today, three African, two Asian and one European type of HP are recognized. In the past, close family groups had their own strain of HP (Enders, 2015).

Rates are higher in developing countries (>75%) and lower in developed countries (<55%). In developing countries, the infection occurs more in children about the age of two to three years and seems to be related to inadequate sanitation, crowded or high density living, and low socio-economic class. Unhygienic food preparation and malnutrition increases risk but adequate nutritional status, eating more fresh fruits and vegetables and increased consumption of vitamin C is protective. This makes sense; you are more likely to pick up an infection when living in poor conditions with inadequate nutrition (Brown, 2000).

HP has coexisted with humans for tens of thousands of years. Since HP has been colonising the human stomach for so many years, is it really hurting us? Could it be a normal commensal? Here we must ask again, if the infection rate is so high, then why doesn't everyone get ulcers? This conundrum needs to be explored.

Even though a very large number of people with

ulcers have been shown to have HP, can it be an important part of our microbiome? Does it provide us with any benefits? The answer is not clear, although there is some evidence to indicate HP has some benefits. Studies have shown that there is an inverse relationship between HP and asthma and allergy. The incidence of asthma started to climb after WW2 in what is considered the start of the antibiotic era. A relationship between asthma and allergy and antibiotics has been noted for some time. Droste et al. (2000) noted that *"Early childhood use of antibiotics is associated with an increased risk of developing asthma and allergic disorders in children who are predisposed to atopic immune responses. These findings support recent immunological understanding of the maturation of the immune system."*

This may not only relate to HP but could also be due to the antibiotics killing off our "good" gut bacteria.

The incidence of HP infections, once high in childhood, has been reducing, possibly because of the frequent use of antibiotics. On the other hand, there has been an increase in the incidence of asthma. Considering the data linking low incidence of HP with asthma and vice versa, is it possible that the rise in asthma in the west is due to increased antibiotic use and thus the reduction in the incidence of HP? The answer, according to Blaser, Chen, and Reibman (2008) is "possibly yes."

As mentioned earlier, children in developing countries, have a high incidence of HP infection, yet they do not often get antibiotics and the incidence of asthma is low (although there may also be other factors involved). Arnold et al. (2011) demonstrated, using a mouse model, that protection against asthma was most robust when HP infection occurred neonatally. This protection was lost when antibiotics were given.

Amedei, Codolo, Del Prete, de Bernard, and D'Elios (2010) showed that HP infection seems to elicit a vigorous Th1 response which can suppress the allergic Th2 response. Th1 is related to cell mediated immunity, while Th2 is related more to antibody related immunity. Of course, it is much more complicated than that, but it seems that HP infection does dampen down an allergic Th2 response.

The connection between the microbiome and the brain has been discussed. Does HP have a role to play?

Budzyński and Kłopocka (2014) demonstrated that there is a gut brain connection involving HP. They state that there is a *bidirectional relationship between HP infection and the brain-gut axis influences both the contagion process and the host's neuroendocrine-immunological reaction to it.*

HP infection should occur in childhood to provide the benefit but due to the frequent use of antibiotics in children in developed countries, HP is eliminated, and asthma and allergy can develop. As the incidence of HP infection has reduced dramatically in the younger age group in developed countries, HP infection may develop in the older age group. However, this older age group does not get the immune benefits of early childhood HP infection, HP in older age groups causes inflammation and possibly leads to ulcers, gastritis, and cancer.

NB: I am not advocating that antibiotics not be used in treating HP. I am saying that the excess use of antibiotics for trivial reasons should stop.

Uemura et al. (2001) demonstrated HP to be a risk factor for stomach cancer. Stomach cancer can be divided into two types depending on the site:

- Cardia cancer (this is the upper part of the stomach, the cardia, where the oesophagus joins the stomach) and
- non-Cardia stomach cancer (i.e., the rest of the stomach).

Hansen, Melby, Aase, Jellum, and Vollset (1999) showed HP to be a risk factor for non-cardia cancer but not cardia cancer. The constant irritation of the stomach by HP is not good. Constant irritation of any cells could lead to cancer. That seems to make sense.

So, why doesn't everyone with HP get ulcers or worse?

One possibility is that HP infection at a young age is beneficial but HP infection at a later age is not.

Another possible reason is that stomach ulcers run in families, so there could be a genetic factor. Yet another possibility is that the strain of HP in that family is more virulent than normal. Certain strains have special genes such as cytotoxin-associated gene A ("CagA") and vacuolating cytotoxin A gene, ("VacA"). If you have any of these strains you are more likely to have stomach problems (Enders, 2015).

Enders, in her book, *Gut* (2015), discusses the connection between HP and PD. She deliberates on the fact that on the island of Guam, there is one area where there is an extraordinarily high proportion of people with Parkinson's-like symptoms. The researchers investigated and found that the inhabitants of this area were eating cycad seeds which have a neurotoxin that can damage the nerves and cause this Parkinson-like disease. As it happens, some strains of HP can produce a very similar neurotoxin. So, what does this mean? Do all people with PD have this strain of HP? Probably not. However, if Parkinson's patients test positive for HP it is a good reason to eliminate HP. Treating HP can improve the PD.

This relationship gets more complicated. Pierantozzi et al. (2001) noted that Parkinson's patients with HP had fluctuating levels of L-dopa (anti-Parkinson's medication) and when the HP was eliminated, they had better control of the disease. They suggested that *"HP infection-activated gastric alterations may be responsible, at least in part, for the reported erratic efficacy of oral L-dopa therapy in some advanced PD patients."*

HP interfered with the absorption of the medication. Lee, Yoon, Shin, Jeon, and Rhee (2008) confirmed this. *"These data demonstrated that HP infection could interfere with the absorption of L-dopa and provoke motor fluctuations. HP eradication can improve the motor fluctuations of HP infected patients with PD."*

To take this even further, there is the Helicobacter hypothesis posited by Dobbs et al. (2008) that HP infection can be part of the cause of PD, or at least involved in the progression of the disease.

Could inflammation be a cause? HP can elicit an inflammatory reaction which can be detected systematically. According to Alvarez-Arellano and Maldonado-Bernal (2014), *"These pro-inflammatory factors can induce brain inflammation and the death of neurons and could eventually be associated to Parkinson's Disease and also may be involved in the development of Alzheimer's Disease."*

It is interesting to point out that there are many gastrointestinal symptoms in the prodrome of PD. Another interesting fact is that the link between gastric ulcers and PD was noted well before HP was even discovered as a cause of ulcers. Ulcers can predate the onset of PD by ten years. Before the discovery of HP and antibiotic treatment, the preferred treatment was surgical; that is, a vagotomy. McGee, Lu, and Disbrow (2018) demonstrated vagotomy to be associated with a decreased risk for PD, suggesting a gut-microbiome-brain link along the Vagus nerve. All Parkinson's patients should be tested for HP. If found, it must be eliminated, whether conventionally with antibiotics, taking into consideration the side effects on the gut microbiome, or using the natural approach that will be discussed in this book.

Smyk et al. (2014) looked at HP antibodies in general and related them to autoimmune diseases, such as Sjogren's syndrome, RA, systemic lupus erythematosus, vasculitides, autoimmune skin conditions, autoimmune thyroid disease, MS, neuromyelitis optica, and autoimmune liver diseases. The researchers discuss the links, correlations, and the strengths of the associations. Some diseases are well studied and have a definite connection, while others are not as well studied, and the results show tenuous links.

More research is needed.

As with PD, check for HP infection in anyone with autoimmune diseases including thyroid disease, especially if there is a history of ulcers or any gut issues. Treating the HP may improve the disease.

Part of the answer to the many unknowns may also be that the problem is not necessarily the bacteria but the immune system. Pasteur is reputed to have said on his deathbed: *"It is the soil, not the seed,"* meaning that it is not only the bacteria that are important when investigating disease, but also the body and competence of the immune system.

What are the factors that allow the bacteria to produce disease?

There are a few facts that are important to know about HP:

- Although HP can survive in an acid environment, its growth and optimal motility is in a more neutral environment. HP is motile between pH 5 and 8, with optimal motility at pH 5. For optimal growth of HP, a pH 6 is needed. The stomach is usually very acidic, around 2-3 (Sidebotham, Worku, Karim, Dhir, & Baron, 2003).
- HP has a protective mechanism which involves an enzyme called *urease.* This enzyme converts urea to alkaline ammonia and therefore

neutralises the acid around it.

- To protect itself further from stomach acid, HP burrows into the mucous layer of the stomach where pH is neutral. It does not enter the epithelial cells but just adheres to them.

- HP releases enzymes *mucinase* and *phospholipase,* as well as toxins, that lead to excess cytokines and chemokines that induces an inflammatory response. This can be seen as gastritis.

- The inflammatory response and the enzymes weaken the mucous layer of the stomach. This breach allows stomach acid to enter and to eat away at the epithelial cells. This mucous layer is the only protection that the stomach has that prevents it digesting itself. This is the start of an ulcer.

It is important to consider that HP grows better in a neutral, or less acidic environment, even though it can survive in a strong acid environment. Why is this important? At the first sign of stomach problems, the initial conventional treatment is an antacid, or some other form of acid suppressing drug. This reduces acid secretion, makes the stomach less acidic, i.e., more alkaline, which makes it a much better environment for HP to grow. Stermer et al. (1997) studied HP positive patients who were divided into two groups. One group was given ranitidine, an acid suppressing drug, and the other group was given a placebo. After two weeks the ranitidine group was shown to have an increased HP bacterial load. Where an acid suppressing drug is used, it could be considered that HP to some extent, is an iatrogenic (doctor-caused) illness.

Giving acid-suppressing drugs can increase
the growth of HP.

As people grow older, the stomach secretes less acid. This can be due to ageing, or stress; this was explored earlier. This makes a lot of elderly people hypochlorhydric, or even achlorhydric, which is a perfect environment for HP to grow.

HP itself can cause enough damage to the acid secreting cells to reduce acid secretion, therefore increasing the chance of growth. Once the HP is eradicated, the stomach can revert to normal acid production, if the damage is not too great.

So, instead of giving acid suppressing drugs, the treatment should be a combination of acid supplements and the other factors mentioned in this book. This keeps the pH low and prevents HP growing.

HP, like other bacteria, develops antibiotic resistance when antibiotics are used indiscriminately. With the indiscriminate use of antibiotics to eradicate HP, antibiotic resistance is developing (Kato et al., 2002).

This will very likely become a big problem in the near future.

HP is developing antibiotic resistance.

How to test for HP

There are 3 main ways to test for HP:

- Urea breath test.
- Blood test for antibodies.
- Faecal antigen test.

Elwyn et al. (2007) compared these three different methods and found that the faecal antigen test was the most effective in terms of true outcomes and cost.

The problem with the blood antibody test is that it cannot differentiate between current or past infections, and so is not a very useful test.

To get over the problems of potential antibiotic resistance and possible biofilm formation, non-antibiotic solutions need to be used. This does not necessarily mean that antibiotics cannot be used. However, if a patient presents with continuing HP infection after one or two or more courses of antibiotic treatment, it is worth changing direction. The saying attributed to Albert Einstein (although there is debate whether Einstein actually said this) is applicable here, *"Insanity is doing the same thing over and over again and expecting a different result."*

Bacteria want to protect themselves, so when they are under frequent antibacterial and/or antibiotic attack, they form biofilms. Then they become harder to eliminate (Zhou, Shi, Huang, & Xie, 2015).

Firstly, the immune system needs to be boosted. There are many ways to do this and one of the best is the use of vitamin C. This is quite fortunate: not only does vitamin C boost the immune system but it is also an effective agent against HP. Simon, Hudes, and Perez-Perez (2003) showed that higher serum levels of ascorbic acid were associated with decreased seroprevalence of HP.

Jarosz et al. (1998) demonstrated a 30% eradication of HP in patients given 5 grams of vitamin C daily for four weeks.

As discussed earlier in the section about biofilms, vitamin C has a quorum sensing inhibiting role, and this may be another reason why vitamin C is beneficial.

Another immune booster and natural antibiotic is garlic. Cañizares et al. (2002) and Sivam (2001) demonstrated that garlic, as well as garlic extracts, are effective against HP. Note that fresh garlic is better than garlic pills.

Another common spice that has been shown to be effective against HP is turmeric (*Curcumin longa*) (Mahady, Pendland, Yun, & Lu, 2002).

García, Salas-Jara, Herrera, and González (2014) showed that curcumin, (the principle curcuminoid of turmeric), has anti-quorum activity against HP. They also comment on the fact that HP can form biofilms in the water distribution system, thus facilitating the spread of the infection. So, other possible vectors are poor sanitation and dirty water in developing countries.

Another natural substance that has shown activity against HP biofilms is N acetylcysteine (NAC). Makipour and Friedenberg (2011) commented that *"Resistance to H. pylori has become increasingly common with triple or quadruple therapy with cure rates of approximately 80%. The success of therapy is thought to be influenced by patient compliance, medication side effects, and antibiotic resistance. A treatment failure rate of 10% to 20% has driven investigators to seek alternative modes of therapy. N-acetylcysteine (NAC), which is capable of destroying bacterial biofilm, is an emerging treatment for recalcitrant infections."*

Even though HP may be a part of the normal microbiome, it can be considered a form of dysbiosis in the context of excess numbers developing at a later age. As one of the treatments for dysbiosis is the use of probiotics, it makes sense that probiotics could help against HP. Wang et al. (2004) demonstrated that the regular intake of yoghurt suppresses HP infections.

The standard treatment for HP is a course or two of antibiotics. Antibiotics may not only kill off the HP in the stomach but also may kill off the "good" bacteria in the gut leading to dysbiosis. So, probiotics are needed not only for replenishing the microbiome, but they may also help with HP eradication. Homan and Orel (2015) noted that *"... specific probiotics, such as S. boulardii and L. johnsonni La1 probably can diminish the bacterial load, but not completely eradicate the H. pylori bacteria."* And *"furthermore, it seems that supplementation with* S. boulardii *is a useful concomitant therapy in the standard* H. pylori *eradication treatment protocol and most probably increases eradication rate. L.* reuteri *is equally effective, but more positive studies are needed. Finally, probiotic strains, such as S. boulardii, L. reuteri and L. GG, decrease gastrointestinal antibiotic associated adverse effects."*

Saccharomyces boulardii is a fungus and is not affected by antibiotics.

The prescription for preventing HP then, is to eat healthy foods, lots of fresh fruits and vegetables high in vitamin C, and eat lots of garlic, yoghurt, and curries. If this is not possible, the next best is to take supplements.

Testing for dysbiosis

Testing for dysbiosis, or any gut problem, requires a specialised test. Although it is the best and most effective test, not all laboratories do the complete digestive stool analysis (CDSA). This is a comprehensive examination of the faeces and looks at biochemical and microbiological parameters of the whole gut from mouth to anus.

Specifically, the CDSA looks at:

- digestion markers,
- absorption markers,
- motility,
- microflora balance,
- metabolic activity, and
- immune function.

The microbiological testing process of the CDSA is different from standard microbiological tests in that the conventional faeces test only looks for bacteria considered pathological. The CDSA looks for the presence and number of bacteria, good, bad, and otherwise, however, it does not test the whole microbiome.

It is an excellent test for assessing the function of the whole gut. The CDSA is more for providing baseline diagnostic information and not specifically for diagnosing underlying conditions, although it can help.

There are other tests that can test your whole microbiome. They may not be cheap but may be useful for treating gut problems where the solution is elusive. A quick internet search can find the various companies that do the test.

Probiotics

To most people, bacteria in the food is a sign that the food is spoiled and rotten and is a cause of disease but there is a group of foods which contain "friendly" bacteria and have health promoting properties.

For centuries, many cultures have used fermented milk products, such as yoghurt, kefir, koumiss, leben and dahi, to stay healthy, and for therapeutic purposes. Beneficial bacteria are also found in fermented foods such as sauerkraut and kimchi and in drinks such as kombucha. Our ancestors did not have refrigerators, so they used fermentation techniques to preserve food.

Modern science is now finding out that the bacteria in these foods do indeed promote better health.

The word "probiotics" comes from the Latin meaning "for life".

Probiotics is defined by the FAO (Food and Agriculture Organization) as *"live micro-organisms administered in adequate amounts which confer a beneficial health effect on the host."*

There are over 400 species of bacteria in the gut, with new species discovered almost daily. The most common probiotics used are the *Lactobacillus* and *Bifidobacterium.* Although the name of some probiotics may be the same as that of some commensals, they are not commensals. As mentioned earlier, probiotics do not replace commensal bacteria, they help to regrow the commensals.

It is well known that our gut is full of bacteria, and we have a symbiotic relationship with them. They are "friendly" bacteria and play a beneficial role in our gut and in our health in general. These bacteria have multiple functions that include:

- helping digestion by producing enzymes, e.g., lactase,
- destroying disease-causing bacteria by producing natural antibiotics,
- keeping Candida in check,
- helping in the production of vitamins, e.g., B complex, vitamin K,
- increasing acidity to make conditions intolerable to dangerous bacteria and
- having a positive effect on the immune function of the gut.

It follows that where there is dysbiosis, part of the treatment is to replace "friendly" bacteria. This can be done by eating foods that contain the bacteria, or by supplementing with a probiotic capsule or powder.

Unless you make your own yoghurt, or similar, there is no guarantee that any product from the supermarket contains adequate live bacteria. Reasons for this is poor food handling, the product may be close to the expiry date, variance of bacteria from batch to batch, and so on.

Despite this, eating these foods does help. Even if you eat yoghurt with dead bacteria, there is some benefit. The cell membranes of these dead bacteria still react with the gut immune system and produce positive effects. A live bacterium is, of course, much better than a dead bacterium.

Probiotics in capsule or powder form are a more definite way to get the bacteria. I recommend that you use capsules or powders and not tablets mainly because in the process of making the tablet, many bacteria are killed.

The studies on probiotics have mixed results. However, there are no negative studies, only some which show benefit and others that show none. Overall, the evidence points to a positive benefit, especially in children (Wanke, 2001).

Probiotics are useful in any gastrointestinal disease, chronic or acute, as well as other conditions such as:

- acute gastroenteritis/food poisoning,

- gut problems after antibiotic use,
- traveller's diarrhoea,
- IBD, such as UC and CrD,
- IBS
- any gut problem,
- dysbiosis,
- possible protection against carcinogens,
- gall bladder disease,
- oestrogen metabolism,
- urogenital/vaginal infections, and
- childhood eczema.

If you go into any health food shop, pharmacy or even supermarket you will find many products with various numbers of bacteria, with various species and strains. It is impossible to say which is the best, however I suggest you choose one with many species and/or strains.

There is growing evidence for the use of specific species or strains for different problems. In a previous discussion EcN was mentioned as being beneficial for chronic constipation. Be aware that each company has their own species/strains and consider it to be the best.

Most useful bacterial strains

So far, the discussion about probiotics has been general. Overall, probiotics/and or fermented foods are beneficial, but studies have looked at different species/strains and investigated whether they are useful for specific conditions. See appendix 3 adapted from Ciorba (2012).

Appendix 3 shows that some probiotics are better than others, depending on what condition you are treating.

It is important to understand that once a probiotic is stopped, it does not stay in the gut for long.

Are there any dangers to taking probiotics? Generally speaking, no, although there may be transient bloating, burping and flatulence.

However, Ciorba (2012) noted that *"Although there are rare cases of bacteremia or fungemia related to the use of probiotics, epidemiologic evidence suggests no population increase in risk on the basis of usage data. There have been many controlled clinical trials on the use of probiotics that demonstrate safe use."* However... *"...a high profile multicenter placebo controlled Dutch*

RCT examining probiotic supplementation in severe acute pancreatitis found a higher incidence of mesenteric ischemia and death in the treatment group. This is the only trial to date to infer such a relationship, but supports the concept that probiotics should be avoided in critically ill patients. Indwelling central vein catheters and perhaps cardiac valvular disease may be relative contraindications."

Basically, probiotics are safe unless you are really sick and are severely immunocompromised.

Prebiotics

Probiotics were discussed earlier but what are prebiotics?

Prebiotics are defined by Gibson et al. (2017) as *"a substrate that is selectively utilized by host microorganisms conferring a health benefit."*

In other words, prebiotics are probiotic food. The gut cannot digest everything and what is not digested is left for the bacteria to use.

Prebiotics are found in a variety of vegetables and fruits which should be part of a healthy diet. These include artichokes, asparagus, tomatoes, onions, garlic, leeks, dandelion greens, spinach, chard, kale, mustard green, legumes, lentils, chickpeas, berries, and bananas.

Breast milk is also a good source of prebiotics and is especially designed for babies, to stimulate the growth of their "friendly" bacteria.

One prebiotic produced on a commercial scale is "fructo oligo saccharides" or FOS. Another prebiotic is "partially hydrolysed guar gum" (PHGG). Both are freely available at any health food shop. SEB can also be considered as a prebiotic. Peterson et al. (2018) showed that SEB (Ulmus rubra) can increase Bifidobacterium, Lactobacillus and Bacteroides species, and specifically reduced potential pathogens such as Citrobacter freundii and Klebsiella pneumoniae. The SEB also increased the relative abundance of butyrate producing bacteria.

Saccharomyces boulardii is a non-pathogenic fungal probiotic but can also act as a prebiotic. Kwak et al. (2022) showed that the oligosaccharides in the cell wall of S. boulardii can function as a prebiotic.

Postbiotics

This is a new concept and Żółkiewicz, Marzec, Ruszczyński, and Feleszko (2020) refer to it as *"any substance released by or produced through the metabolic activity of the microorganism, which exerts a beneficial effect on the host, directly or indirectly."* This includes short-chain-fatty-acids (SCFA), exopolysaccharides, enzymes, cell wall fragments, cell-free supernatants (a mixture of compounds produced by bacteria and yeast) and various other metabolites such as vitamins and amino acids.

Postbiotic supplements are not widely available at present, so the best way to increase postbiotics is to supplement prebiotics and probiotics.

Leaky gut syndrome (LGS)

"It is more important to know what sort of patient has the disease than to know what sort of disease has the patient."
William Osler (1849-1919)

LGS is a concept that involves the idea that the gut, being a semi-permeable membrane, becomes more permeable when damaged and allows molecules to gain access into the body that normally would not be allowed.

The definition of the LGS is *"A gastrointestinal tract dysfunction caused by increased permeability of the intestinal wall, which allows absorption of toxic material, bacteria, fungi, parasites etc; LGS may be linked to allergy and various autoimmune conditions."* (*McGraw-Hill Concise Dictionary of Modern Medicine* (2002). Retrieved April 24, 2023)

A natural assumption about our GI system is that it can, and should, control what enters the body. The semi-permeable nature of the gut is not random. There is some form of control, which when considered, makes a lot of sense. It is not helpful to allow any and every molecule to enter our body indiscriminately. Our GI system is designed so that there is selective absorption of some molecules but not others. It is the cells that line the lumen of the gut and the tight junctions between them that have the task of selecting what is absorbed and what is not.

In the healthy gut, this control is optimal and is a finely tuned mechanism. This finely tuned system breaks down when there is damage to these cells and/or when the tight junction between the cells is loosened. When this happens, molecules, toxins, and peptides, which normally do not get into the body, can get into the body and cause disease and damage.

Many of the symptoms of LGS do not necessarily refer to the gut itself. The poor digestion, the dysbiosis, the food allergies or insensitivities, the chemicals in the diet that cause the symptoms of bloating, gurgling, pain, constipation, or diarrhoea, are all factors that cause the gut to become leaky, not LGS itself. Essentially, anything that can cause gut damage can also cause LGS.

The symptoms of LGS can be much more global. The following conditions have been linked to LGS: asthma, autoimmune diseases, chronic joint pain, chronic muscle pain, confusion, fuzzy or foggy thinking, mood swings, nervousness, poor immunity, recurrent vaginal infections, skin rashes, bed wetting, recurrent bladder infections, poor memory, shortness of breath, aggressive behaviour, anxiety, fatigue and "feeling toxic."

Mainstream medicine does not necessarily agree with all of this, although according to Aleman, Moncada, and Aryana (2023) some are starting to accept the concept. Also, it is becoming evident that the connection between LGS and autoimmunity is more accepted by mainstream practitioners.

It is important to understand the connection between leaky gut, molecular mimicry, and autoimmune diseases. A healthy gut does not allow molecules, peptides, toxins, etc., into the body; a leaky gut does. These molecules, peptides, and toxins can be regarded by the body as "foreign" and it reacts to them accordingly, with an immunological response, antibody formation and B cell response. If some of these molecules are structurally similar to human "self" molecules, then the antibodies made, can cross react with "self" molecules. This is the concept of molecular mimicry and the start of autoimmunity (Cusick, Libbey, & Fujinami, 2012; Paray, Albeshr, Jan, & Rather, 2020).

Causes of LGS

Anything that can damage the gut mucosa can cause LGS. Damage can be caused by a large variety of factors:

- Stress. The cells that line the intestine have a fast turn-over rate; they replace themselves approximately every two to five days. To do this, they need a very good blood supply. The gut is probably the first area that loses its normal blood supply with the "flight and flight" reaction. Therefore, stress has a great impact upon the function of the gut. Poor blood supply = poor nourishment of the cells = poor function of the cells.
- Various foods such as gluten, alcohol, caffeine, cocoa, chocolate, and various soft drinks such as cola, can irritate the gut mucosa and therefore interfere with its function.
- Food contaminated with various bacteria. This is related to dysbiosis which we have already discussed. Also, hypochlorhydria, where there is a lack of stomach acid to kill off any micro-organisms in the food we eat.
- Chemicals in food, either purposefully added, such as colourings, flavours, and preservatives,

or unintentionally added such as contaminants, insecticides, pesticides, etc. This is like the second point. The difference is that the chemicals in the food are naturally found in these foods. Unfortunately, manufacturers add many different chemicals to foods to assist in taste, colour and for preservation. Other chemicals found in food are pollutants which is becoming a more and more serious problem.

- Diet high in sugars, carbohydrates, especially white bread, and other highly refined products. These foods encourage the growth of yeasts, such as Candida and other dysbiotic bacteria and parasites.
- Antibiotics, which kill off the "good" bacteria and promote overgrowth of yeasts and "bad" bacteria. We have already explored this with dysbiosis.
- Other drugs, such as non-steroidal anti-inflammatory NSAIDs, steroids, hormones, etc.
- Food allergies and insensitivities. This is probably the greatest cause of LGS and unfortunately is not generally recognised. Food allergy is recognised but not food intolerances. This will be the focus of discussion in another section. There is dairy allergy and gluten allergy (also known as CD), which is recognised but, unfortunately, the grey areas are not recognised,

the dairy and gluten intolerance, and these probably account for most of the cases.

- Methylation problems, as already discussed.

Many people confuse, or even conflate, allergy and intolerance (toxicity). It is important to differentiate between them. Dairy allergy and gluten allergy are well known. Gluten allergy is known as CD. However, intolerance to dairy and gluten falls into a "grey area" and is not generally recognised by mainstream practitioners. Unfortunately, intolerance to foods containing gluten and dairy probably accounts for most of the cases where patients struggle with the symptoms outlined above.

It is standard medical practice to perform blood tests and/or skin prick tests to detect allergies. With dairy and gluten intolerance, the tests are invariably negative. The patients are reassured that there is no dairy or gluten allergy. In the strict sense, this is true, there is no allergy but there is still a problem. The person may not be allergic to that food, but there is an intolerance. In other words, the food doesn't like the person.

I have met many people, and you probably know people like this, who struggle through life. They are tired and sluggish; their abdomens bloat up and their bowels are problematic. They may not be sick, but they are not well either. They struggle on; they accept this fate that life has given them. They do not know better. How many people do you know who are like this? You may even be one of them.

These are people who probably have a food intolerance and, as you probably have guessed, the worst offenders are the grains (especially the gluten fraction) and dairy.

My first advice to anyone like this is to stop dairy and grains. It is surprising how many respond positively; their energy improves, their abdominal bloating is reduced, and their bowel actions normalise. If stopping these foods does not make any difference, then there must be some other issue.

> "Food intolerance is like hitting your head against the wall. You only know how good it feels when you stop!"

Many people worry that they will miss out on nutrients because they believe that these foods are beneficial. "Where do I get my calcium from?" is a very common question when I advise people to stop dairy. These two foods groups are not essential for human health. Patients are reassured to know that vegetables such as cauliflower, broccoli, and nuts are a good source of calcium.

Those who are suffering have spent a lifetime adhering to advice that they should drink their milk and eat their bread and pasta, not knowing it may be doing them harm.

From a historical perspective, dairy and grains have been a part of the human diet for less than 10,000 years. Although that sounds a very long time, the human species has lived on this planet for much longer. In fact, the amount of time our species has been eating these foods is far less than the time we did not eat them. Our genes change very slowly, we still have "caveman" genes, we are adapted to a "caveman" diet. Overall, despite some people not reacting to these foods, most have not adapted to grains and dairy, which were never a part of the cave man diet. Essentially, it is up to the individual. Regardless of whether the experts, or this book, says to eat a particular food, if it makes you feel unwell, don't eat it.

Our metabolism is more adapted to a "hunter-gatherer" diet, not an agricultural diet.

I can hear howls of protest. Yes, it is possible to survive on an agricultural diet, and some will manage better than others. However, while there are some people who can better tolerate these foods, there are also many who cannot; while these people are not sick, neither are they well.

So, while it is possible to survive on these foods (it is better than starving) this does not necessarily mean that they allow us to achieve our maximum genetic potential.

One theory is that we had no choice. As the population grew and the number of animals to hunt declined, something had to be done, otherwise our species may have starved into extinction. We had to survive on this agricultural diet but is it the best for us? Some sections of the population seem to have adapted well but a significant number have not.

This pre-amble has introduced the idea that dairy and grains are not necessarily the best foods for some of us. I had a patient once who was a wheat farmer and he told me, *"I grow the stuff... but I don't eat it!!"*

As mentioned, the two main foods that can cause problems are gluten, which is found in wheat and more specifically grains, and dairy. These foods can cause bowel problems leading to LGS.

During the normal course of events food that is eaten is digested: proteins are broken down into individual amino acids that the body can absorb. If digestion is faulty, the breakdown is incomplete. The bowel contains many other things, such as bacteria, Candida, toxins from these organisms and substances that would not be healthy if they entered the body.

Normally, these gut contents do not enter the body, but with LGS, these substances may do so through damaged cells and loosened, normally tight, junctions between the cells.

For example, if proteins are injected intravenously, death will occur. If we inject amino acids, there is no problem, so proteins need to be completely digested to their amino acid components.

With LGS, partly digested proteins, peptides of varying sizes, are able to enter the body. So too may bacteria or bacterial proteins. Toxins may also enter. The body treats these substances the same way it treats all foreign proteins; the immune system detects them, labels them as foreign and an immune reaction is started. Antibodies may be made against these substances. This can be the start of food allergies, auto-immune diseases, and other diseases (Rojas et al., 2018; Fasano, 2012).

Testing for LGS

If we are serious about detecting and treating LGS, we must be able to test for it and then, and only then, can we assess the success of our treatment.

There is a very simple test and as for other disorders, only certain laboratories perform it.

Intestinal permeability can be assessed by the dual sugar technique. This involves giving an oral dose of two sugars, mannitol, and lactulose. Mannitol is readily absorbed by passive transport into the intestinal cells, (mean absorption 14%, range 5-25%) while lactulose is virtually not absorbed by the normal gut (less than 1%). These sugars are not metabolised by the gut and what is absorbed is quickly excreted in the urine after six hours.

By giving a known quantity of these sugars orally and then examining the urine for them, the intestinal permeability can be determined. In a normal gut the lactulose/mannitol ratio is 0.03, i.e., mannitol is easily absorbed, lactulose is not.

The higher the ratio, the greater the lactulose absorption, therefore the leakier the gut.

In this way, intestinal permeability can be assessed and monitored.

Treating LGS

There are three perspectives to be considered in the treatment of LGS (or any other gut disease).

First, elimination (removal) of the factors that caused, or are thought to have caused, the problem in the first place.

Second, supplementing (replacing) what is missing in the gut with what it needs to function properly.

Third, repairing any damage.

The 3 Rs – Remove, Replace, Repair.

There are variations on this theme:

3 Rs Remove, Repair, and Reinoculate.

4 Rs Remove, Replace, Reinoculate and Repair. To reinoculate is to replace the microbiome with probiotics.

So far, the first and second points have been discussed.

In summary, the goal is to eliminate the underlying cause. Therefore, certain foods, such as dairy and grains, and perhaps any other food which is causing an allergy or intolerance must be eliminated. As well, dysbiosis or any parasitic infection must be treated. Then those things that the gut needs, such as acid, digestive enzymes, prebiotics and probiotics are provided through supplementation.

The third point is to repair any damage. To do this, the body must be fed properly.

Of course, there is a long list of things that can be done but as some are more important than others, these will be the focus of the following discussion.

Glutamine

L-Glutamine is an amino acid that is classified as a "non-essential" amino acid. This means that the body can make it, but during times of stress, injury, or infection, there is a glutamine deficiency. Glutamine is needed for energy and is the most ideal nutrient for the regeneration of enterocytes, the cells that line the intestines. Enterocytes are the only cells in the body that do not obtain their nutrition from the blood but directly from the contents of the intestines. Glutamine is an abundant amino acid in both plant and animal protein. The typical American diet supplies 3.5 to 7.0 grams a day and more is synthesised if needed.

Glutamine has multiple functions in the brain, in muscles, and in maintaining blood sugar levels. As far as the gut is concerned, glutamine is the preferred food for the cells that line the intestines. A well-fed cell works very much better than a poorly fed cell. Intestinal cells have a high turnover rate and are metabolically very active. They need to be well fed. Glutamine also has a beneficial effect on the liver and can protect the liver from damage.

A useful supplement for any gut disease, glutamine is not only helpful for treating LGS, or diarrhoea, but also is effective as an adjunct therapy in the treatment of UC and CD. It has also been found to aid in protecting the mucosa from the damaging effects of NSAIDS and chemotherapy. Doses can range from 2-3 grams for mild disease to 20 grams a day in serious illnesses (Zhou et al., 2019; Achamrah, Déchelotte, & Coëffier, 2017).

Zinc

Zinc is found in all cells of the body and is a major co-factor for at least 150 enzymes. Zinc is an important mineral in intestinal wall integrity and contributes to the healing of the leaky gut. It also maintains a healthy immune system.

Zinc supplementation in CD was shown to improve the lactulose/mannitol ratio by improving the leaky gut (Sturniolo, Di Leo, Ferronato, D'Odorico, & D'Incà, 2001).

Meat, especially beef, is the richest source of zinc known, so therefore, you need to eat meat (refer to the section on DD where the eating of meat is discussed). This is becoming a problem because it is trendy to eat less meat, although the recent popularity of the Paleo diet, the ketogenic diet and, of course, the Atkins Diet, is reversing the trend to some extent. Meat eating needs to be in the "Goldilocks' zone"; not too much, not too little.

There is a very close relationship between protein and zinc. Insufficient protein intake may cause a zinc deficiency. Zinc deficiency predisposes to poor immune function, causing an overgrowth of toxin-producing bacteria, or enteroviruses that can produce diarrhoea, which can exacerbate the already compromised mineral status. The gastrointestinal tract may be one of the first target areas when zinc deficiency is manifested (Wapnir, 2000).

Zinc can be supplemented using 15-30 mg daily.

Dr Peter Baratosy MBBS FACNEM

Slippery elm bark (SEB)

SEB comes from the inner bark of a tree (*Ulmus rubra* and *Ulmus fulva*) that grows in North America. It has been used for centuries in traditional medicine to treat sore throats, wounds and to ease digestive disorders.

The bark is very rich in mucilage, a mixture of polysaccharides that becomes gelatinous when mixed with water. This "mucous" is very soothing and helps to reduce inflammation. It can be used externally, e.g., inflamed skin conditions, or internally, to sooth the inflamed gastrointestinal tract from mouth to anus.

The mucilage has other beneficial properties. It:

- reduces bowel transit time,
- absorbs toxins from the bowel,
- increases faecal bulk,
- dilutes faecal materials and reduces stool contact with intestinal mucosa,
- enhances beneficial bacteria in the gut (prebiotic), and
- sooths inflamed gastrointestinal mucosa.

The mucilage resists gastric acid and enzymes and therefore retains its action throughout the whole gut. This herb is a wonderful healing agent for any gastrointestinal problem (Ried, Travica, Dorairaj, & Sali, 2020).

There are many other nutrients that can be supplemented, including vitamins A C, and E, fish oils, other antioxidants, and many others. These can be used if, and when, needed.

Molecular mimicry

"Man is a food dependant creature; if you don't feed him, he will die. If you feed him improperly, part of him will die."
Emanuel Cheraskin (1916-2001)

"Molecular mimicry or "molecular similarity" is an important concept in immunology and immunotoxicology, whereby external antigens that resemble some "self-antigens" will lead to an immune response which will cause tissue damage to the host, and this is called autoimmunity" (Ebringer, Hughes, Rashid, & Wilson, 2005).

The antigen can be a foreign protein from a virus, a bacterium, even a vaccine (Segal & Shoenfeld, 2018). This foreign protein can also be from the (partial) digestion of some foods, notably dairy and grains, although it could be from any food. As discussed above, LGS is part of this process. A normal gut will not allow these molecules to enter the body.

There is evidence that auto-immune diseases such as MS, RA, CD, type 1 diabetes (T1D), atherosclerosis and perhaps others are related to molecular mimicry (Rojas et al., 2018; Kukreja & Maclaren, 2000). The rubella virus and a coxsackie virus have been implicated in diabetes but the main culprits involved in molecular mimicry are food proteins, mainly grains (especially the gluten component) and dairy (casein: the protein of milk). The geographical distribution of diseases, such as MS and T1D follows a pattern of food habits rather than differences in infectious agents.

The process is that people eat these foods, the proteins are partially digested to peptides of varying lengths, which are then absorbed through the "leaky gut." The body recognises the peptides as foreign and therefore mounts an immunological reaction against them. This is a case of "mistaken identity." These antibodies cross-react with various tissues such as beta islets of the pancreas (T1D), joint cartilage (RA) and the lining of the arteries (arteriosclerosis).

Anti-gliadin antibodies (AGA) are the hallmark of CD but are also encountered in IgA nephritis, psoriasis, sickle cell anaemia, hepatic disorders, juvenile RA, autoimmune thyroiditis, and in persons who occupationally come into contact with great amounts of wheat. *"The emergence of AGA in immunomediated diseases may be attributed to the response to food protein in pathological conditions and is often unrelated closely with Coeliac Disease"* (Kamaeva, Reznikov, Pimenova, & Dobritsyna, 1998).

As mentioned earlier, these foods have only relatively recently been introduced into the human diet and are the main problem for those with food allergies and sensitivities. Molecular mimicry provides another good reason to avoid these foods, especially if you suffer from diabetes, RA, or MS, or even if there is a family history of these diseases.

Dr Peter Baratosy MBBS FACNEM

Ankylosing spondylitis

It is well accepted in orthodox circles that the antigen HLA-B27 is linked to ankylosing spondylitis (AS). It has been shown that there is a similarity between HLA-B27 and *nitrogenase* and *pullulanase D*, which are two enzymes from a bacterial species called Klebsiella, which is involved in dysbiosis. We can speculate that these enzymes from the dysbiotic bowel are absorbed through the leaky gut and the body reacts to them and then cross reacts with the HLA-B27.

Rheumatoid arthritis

RA is a complex multi-factorial disease which has environmental and genetic factors. Just as AS is linked to HLA-B27, RA is linked to HLA-DR1/DR4. Again, there is a similarity between HLA-DR1/DR4 and *haemolysin* which is a molecule from a bacterial species called *Proteus,* which is also involved in dysbiosis.

A dietary connection has also been made. In fact, two staple western foods have been implicated.

Dairy proteins have been implicated. Residues 141-157 of bovine albumin was significantly different from human albumin but was highly homologous with human collagen type 1. This would suggest a molecular mimicry mechanism for RA and dairy products (Pérez-Maceda, López-Bote, Langa, & Bernabeu,1991).

There is enough evidence to implicate the gluten fraction of grains in the development of RA. Grains are a very prominent part of the western diet. Anecdotal evidence indicates that fasting and/or grain elimination from the diet improves the clinical course of RA (Hafström et al., 2001).

Of course, not everyone who eats dairy and wheat contracts RA. Since RA is a complex interplay between genetics and environment, there is possibly only a sub-group that reacts to these foods. Conversely, if you have RA, it is worth trying dairy and wheat elimination. It may positively impact the course of the disease.

Multiple sclerosis

It has been well established that many viruses and bacteria have amino acid sequences that resemble sequences in the myelin of the central nervous system. A sequence of proteins found on the surface of the hepatitis B virus has a similar sequence to proteins found in myelin, the lipid substance that forms a sheath around nerve fibres.

Hepatitis B infections are known to be associated, although rarely, with:

- central nervous system demyelinating disease (Santos-García, Arias-Rivas, Dapena, & Arias, 2007),
- transverse myelitis (Iñiguez et al., 2000; Basheer, Mookkappan, Shanmugham, & Natarajan, 2014),
- optic neuritis (Galli, Morelli, Casellato, & Perna,1986), and
- Guillain-Barre syndrome (Yimam, Merriman, & Todd Frederick, 2013).

Could these be other instances of molecular mimicry?

There are also food proteins that have similar sequences. Research of MS geographical distribution follows differences in dietary habit rather than infections, and the usual suspects are again wheat and dairy (Agranoff & Goldberg, 1974; Shor et al., 2009).

According to Hernández-Lahoz and Rodrigo (2013) and Rodrigo et al. (2014) going gluten free and dairy free may help with MS.

Diabetes type 1

T1D, also known as insulin dependent diabetes mellitus, (IDDM) develops when the beta cells of the pancreas, which are the cells that manufacture insulin, are attacked by antibodies. Where do these antibodies come from? It is evident that molecular mimicry and various proteins may be involved. A protein from the coxsackie virus has been implicated: there is a cross reaction with the p2C protein of the coxsackie virus and a protein in the beta cells of the pancreas (Vreugdenhil et al., 1998).

This is not necessarily true for all type 1 diabetics. The paper indicates that it may only be limited to the HLA-DR3 positive sub-group.

Cows' milk can trigger diabetes in at-risk children. Virtanen et al. (1994), Gerstein and VanderMeulen (1996) and Saukkonen et al. (1998) showed a strong relationship between cow's milk exposure and IDDM.

Virtanen et al. (1994) showed that IDDM-prone children who were breast fed in the first months of life were less likely to develop IDDM than similar at-risk children who were fed on cows' milk-based formula. Antibodies to a bovine serum albumin peptide were found in 100% of recently diagnosed early onset diabetics, while it was hardly ever found in normal controls.

Coeliac disease (CD)

"What is food to one, is to others bitter poison."
Lucretius (96 BC- 55 BC)

CD is a genetic disease where there is a "true" allergy to gluten, a protein component of grain (includes wheat, barley, oats, rye and spelt). The most important genes are HLA DQ2 and HLA DQ8. Most people with CD have these genes. The carrier rate of these genes is 30% but only 1 in 30 gets CD. Having the gene doesn't automatically mean a 100% chance of getting CD, so it must not be a fully genetic disease; there must be some environmental triggers. If a first degree relative has CD, you have a 10% chance of getting it. In identical twins there is only a 70% concomitant rate.

This is not the full story. There are hidden factors that at present are still being investigated. The story started in Sweden in the mid-1980s where a huge spike in CD developed. The rate among the babies quadrupled. This 'epidemic' lasted until about the mid-1990s and did not happen in any other neighbouring country.

Why?

What happened?

Researchers have been looking at this and the full reason has not been elucidated, though there are a few clues. In the mid-80s there was a change in infant feeding; breast feeding was down to 50% at six months and the popularity of "follow on" formula was increasing. These formulae were thickened with wheat flour, so the intake of gluten almost doubled during the mid-80s, with the babies suddenly getting a huge hit of gluten. By the mid-90s the feeding practices had changed. "Follow on" formulae usage declined, and therefore the gluten intake declined. Breastfeeding rates increased, and the advice was to introduce gluten slowly between four and six months of age.

The whole issue is still confusing, but it is safe to say:

- do not introduce gluten too early, e.g., before 4 months of age, although as will be discussed later, it is even better if gluten is not introduced in the first 12 months,
- introduce gluten slowly, and
- breastfeed.

If there is a strong family history of CD then it would be wise to be even more careful. Before introducing gluten, do genetic testing.

There are still other possible environmental factors that have not been discovered. The prevalence of CD has increased 4-5-fold in USA, Finland, and the UK over the last 50 years, but the presence of HLA genotypes and the gluten content of wheat has not changed. Ludvigsson and Green (2014) identified other factors, or at least considered them, such as elective Caesarean section, perinatal and childhood infections, use of antibiotics and use of PPIs.

As well, during this "epidemic' the ratio of boys to girls developing CD was about 1:2. Outside of the "epidemic" period the ratio was about 1:1, so girls seem to have been genetically more sensitive to environmental exposure, whatever it may have been (Ivarsson, Persson, Nyström, & Hernell, 2003).

Another study showed that the highest risk was in children who had several infections before six months of age, had eaten large amounts (as compared to small or medium amounts) of gluten, and for whom breastfeeding was stopped before introduction of the gluten (Myléus et al., 2012).

Kahrs et al. (2019) demonstrated that in coeliac genotype carrying children, an enterovirus infection during childhood can trigger CD later in life, while an adenovirus infection does not.

So, at this stage, there is no way of knowing for sure what all the factors are. You need the genes, but you also need an environmental trigger.

In CD there is an actual allergy to gluten: antibodies to gluten are found in the blood, although they do disappear on a gluten free (GF) diet. This allergy causes intestinal damage. Even though it is a genetic disorder, to manifest itself, it must have an environmental trigger and as mentioned above, gluten in the diet is not the only factor.

Initially, gluten allergy was thought to be quite rare, occurring as infrequently as 1 in 5,000. However, Hill et al. (2000) showed CD to be more common than previously thought. In a group of children with GI symptoms, the researchers found an incidence of 1 in 57, and it could have been as high as 1 in 33. This, of course is amongst a selected group of symptomatic children.

An earlier study by Ivarsson, Hernell, Stenlund, and Persson (2002) showed that breastfeeding was protective from developing CD while introducing gluten containing foods. The risk of CD was reduced in the group of children who were breastfed and were starting on gluten containing foods compared to a group that was not breast fed. This same study also showed that slow introduction of small amounts of gluten containing foods reduced the risk of CD as compared to fast introduction of large amounts.

However, the findings of a 2014 study by Lionetti et al. did not concur. According to the results of this study, breastfeeding is extremely beneficial for the baby but there does not seem to be any protection from CD. The study results also disproved the "window of safety" theory that suggests gluten can be introduced safely between four and six months. This study showed that it doesn't matter when gluten is introduced, and it doesn't matter if you breast feed, you will still get CD if you have the HLA genotype. However, this study did show that if gluten is introduced at a later age there is a delayed onset of the disease.

CD can also present in other ways and the interesting thing is that there does not necessarily have to be GI symptoms. Duggan (2004) referred to CD as the "great imitator" of the 20th Century. In the past, syphilis was referred to as the great imitator, but this disease is virtually unseen today.

Duggan (2004) showed that CD can present as, or be associated with:

- **Gastrointestinal problems:** Liver disease, "transaminitis", hepatitis, fatty liver, primary biliary cirrhosis, cirrhosis, recurrent aphthous mouth ulcers, "irritable bowel syndrome", lymphocytic gastritis, ulcerative jejunitis, reflux oesophagitis, adenocarcinoma of the small bowel.

Case Study

A 16-year-old girl, known to have CD presented with recurrent mouth ulcers and some recurrence of gut pains indicating that she was having gluten from some source. A thorough diet history showed no obvious exposure. In conjunction with her parents, we had a long, hard think about where she could possibly be encountering gluten. Finally, it dawned on us. She was 16 with a new boyfriend. Surely there is some saliva exchange at some point. The advice given was that the boyfriend must be gluten free before there was to be any more kissing. The new boyfriend complied, and she did settle after that!

- **Neurological problems**: Peripheral neuropathy, epilepsy, ataxia, myelopathy, in fact any neurological condition of unknown origin. Hadjivassiliou et al. (2002) showed that anti-gliadin antibodies cross-react with Purkinje cells in the cerebellum causing gluten ataxia.

Case Study

Mr KH aged 35 presented with sudden onset of seizures. He was fully investigated in the hospital; CT scan, MRI, and EEG were all normal. There was no family history of epilepsy, no past history of head trauma. The hospital wanted to medicate him with anti-epileptic drugs. He refused. I saw him and on taking his history he gave a history of gut pain and bloating, especially when he ate bread. Remember that CD can present with any neurological condition of unknown origin. So, I checked his coeliac serology, and it was very high. He refused endoscopy and biopsy; he was happy just to know that he more than likely had CD. He stopped gluten 100%. The seizures disappeared and he made a full recovery, which continues if he remains totally gluten free.

- **Psychiatric problems**: Depression, schizophrenia.
- **Endocrine problems**: T1D, infertility in men and women, recurrent abortions, thyroid disorders, Addison's disease.

Case Study

A 19-year-old young lady presented with a history of hyperthyroidism. This was complicated by the fact that she was also allergic to carbimazole and propylthiouracil (PTU), the two available medications used to treat hyperthyroidism. The hyperthyroidism settled spontaneously in February 2018. She presented to me in November 2018 with recurrence of symptoms typical of hyperthyroidism; tremor, weight loss, palpitations, feeling hot, etc. despite her thyroid function test (TFT) showing only a slight thyroid stimulating hormone (TSH) suppression with normal T3 and T4.

She was seeing the endocrinologist who had referred her to a surgeon with a view of thyroidectomy. She came to me for another opinion. A significant part of her history was that she was very iron deficient and iron supplementation was not very helpful. Family history included two cousins with CD. I tested her coeliac antibodies, and they were very high, consistent with CD. She refused endoscopy and biopsy. She stopped gluten and immediately felt better. Being a coeliac, oral iron supplements would be useless, so I arranged for an iron infusion.

At this early stage I cannot say if the hyperthyroidism will totally settle, or whether she will eventually need a thyroidectomy. Research shows a strong relationship between CD and autoimmune thyroid disease, mainly hypothyroidism although hyperthyroidism can occur less frequently. Treating the CD by totally going gluten free may resolve the hyperthyroidism therefore preventing a thyroidectomy.

A subsequent TFT was normal. Follow up continues.

Freeman (2016) studied 96 adults with recently confirmed CD, which revealed 16 with autoimmune thyroid disease. All had hypothyroidism although of these, four previously had Graves' Disease and had already been treated with thyroidectomy or radioactive iodine. Theoretically, if CD was diagnosed earlier, they may still have their thyroid.

- **Renal problems**: IgA nephropathy.
- **Haemopoietic problems**: Anaemia (iron, folate and vitamin B12 deficiency), coagulation disorders from vitamin K deficiency, IgA deficiency, hyposplenism, T-cell lymphoma.

Case Study

A young lady presented to me with tiredness. I did routine blood tests and found she was anaemic and had a low iron. She did complain of heavy periods. I started her on iron supplements and the herb vitex agnus castus for the heavy periods, assuming the heavy periods were the cause of her anaemia. On follow up there was minimal change to her iron levels. After some thought, I checked her coeliac serology, and the antibodies were high. She had the endoscopy and biopsy which confirmed CD. She is now 100% gluten free and has no more iron deficiency problems.

- **Locomotor problems**: Arthralgia/arthritis, osteopoenia.
- **Dermatological problems**: Dermatitis herpetiformis, psoriasis, brown pigmentation of face and buccal mucosa.
- **Dental problems**: Defects in tooth enamel.
- **Genetic problems**: Down's syndrome.
- **Cardiovascular problems**: Cardiomyopathy.
- **Other**: Alopecia areata, Sjogren's syndrome, systemic lupus erythematosus (SLE), fatigue, finger clubbing, pharangeal and oesophageal carcinoma.

Note. CD is an autoimmune disease. If you have one autoimmune disease, you are prone to develop other autoimmune diseases.

Case Study

A 30-year-old gentleman presented with a long history of mild gastrointestinal discomfort, mild tiredness and just mildly feeling unwell. All in all, every one of his symptoms was described as "mild" and he lived his life to the fullest but all the time "just not feeling well".

On the first consultation, he pulled a pile of papers, about one and a half inches thick, out of his bag and plonked it on my desk "These", he said "are all the tests that have been done!" Since we were limited in time, I quickly went through all the tests, blood tests, x-rays, urine tests, poo tests, saliva tests. You name it, it was there. All were normal, or only just mildly abnormal, mild liver enzyme elevation and mild iron deficiency. I started treating him with my usual supplements and after a few months, there was no improvement. He had been on a GF diet and no improvement. I was confused and didn't know where to go next. So, I asked him to bring back all his tests again and I had a much closer look. Again, all normal or only mildly abnormal. Then it dawned on me; as Sherlock Holmes once noted, it is the absence of something that may be the clue. The one test that wasn't done was a coeliac test.

I ordered coeliac serology, and it came back positive. He had CD. In retrospect, his GF diet was not 100% and only half hearted. So, once the diagnosis was made and he started a strict gluten free diet, he improved greatly.

10-18% of patients present primarily with anaemia, 20% with tiredness and 43% with malabsorption and bowel symptoms.

Essentially, anyone who is suffering from any of the above diseases needs to be investigated for CD and if CD is found and treated, the presenting disease can be improved and even cured. The treatment is relatively simple; totally avoid gluten.

Dr Peter Baratosy MBBS FACNEM

Gluten intolerance

As mentioned earlier, there are people who do not have CD but who do have gluten intolerance, otherwise known as non-coeliac gluten sensitivity (NCGS). The difference is that gluten intolerance is not based on an allergy to gluten. Those with NCGS may have similar symptoms as CD but there is no evidence of any damage to the small intestine villi. There are no anti-gliaden antibodies. Gluten intolerance is a clinical diagnosis, based on clinical symptoms of abdominal bloating, generally feeling unwell and tiredness as well as a negative coeliac test. A trial of a gluten free diet can give dramatic results. Another way to look at it is; if the clinical symptoms fit but the blood tests are normal then it probably is NCGS. It is a diagnosis of exclusion.

This is the main reason why anyone with gut symptoms has been advised to avoid wheat (gluten). Naturopaths and nutritional doctors have been giving this advice for years. Many with gut problems do feel better after stopping wheat and other gluten containing grains. Certainly, a trial of a gluten free (GF) diet is worthwhile. I generally would recommend a GF diet if there were any history of gut problems. However, as will be discussed later, gluten can affect a normal gut.

So, who should go on a gluten free diet?

In my opinion those who should avoid gluten are:

- anyone with CD, no ifs or buts,
- anyone who feels sick or unwell when eating gluten containing foods. However, it is important to note the cause may not necessarily be the gluten. There are other things in breads, pasta, and cereals besides gluten that may cause gut problems, e.g., FODMAPs. From a practical point of view, if you feel unwell eating a particular food, then don't eat it!

There are people who do not get sick or unwell from eating these foods but still choose not to eat gluten. This may be a fad or there may be other personal reasons. Not eating gluten foods does not do any harm. Although one important thing to stress is that while not eating gluten containing foods, it is essential to still eat properly; eggs, meat, fish, vegetables, salads, nuts, seeds, fruits, and so on. You do not necessarily need a substitute for the gluten containing foods.

Gluten free (GF) products can be more expensive and not very tasty or healthy, so is necessary to be discerning about what you choose to buy. New GF products taste much better.

Many GF products use rice flour as the substitute and research shows that rice products can contain high levels of arsenic. Rice is known to bioaccumulate heavy metals such as arsenic and mercury. An unintended consequence of a gluten free diet can be arsenic toxicity (Bulka, Davis, Karagas, Ahsan, & Argos, 2017).

Rice cakes are the worst! The Swedish National Food Agency recommends not giving rice cakes to children under the age of six. Boiling rice and then draining off the water can reduce the arsenic content by half. The issue is with people eating GF products in large amounts because of the high rice content consumed.

In a 2014 study carried out by Rahman, Rahman, Reichman, Lim, and Naidu, Australian grown rice was shown to have a higher arsenic content than rice imported from Asia, although less than the standards set by Food Standards Australia and New Zealand (Fransisca et al., 2015).

Daily rice consumption increases the chance of arsenic toxicity, so it is wise to comply with the Swedish National Food Agency's recommendations to eat rice less frequently (Swedish National Food Agency 2015).

While there may not be an acute arsenic toxicity, long-term rice eating may cause chronic arsenic poisoning. This could lead to cancer and other conditions such as skin changes, hyperpigmentation, headaches, drowsiness, confusion, peripheral neuropathy, peripheral vasculopathy and more.

Also, as mentioned, rice can bio-accumulate mercury. Zhang, Feng, Larssen, Qiu, and Vogt (2010) showed that in inland China, rice rather than fish is the major reason for methylmercury exposure.

For whatever reason, mainstream medicine is very against GF diets. They maintain that only CD sufferers need to be off gluten. Their concerns emanate, they say, from the damage that missing out on certain food groups may cause.

Gluten production by plants is a defence mechanism. Since plants cannot run away, they make gluten to cause stomach-ache in animals, which discourages animals from eating them. The animals learn not to eat that plant.

Numerous people with gut complaints stop eating gluten because they feel better.

How <u>dare</u> they feel better by not eating gluten!

Added to this, for very similar reasons, a dairy free (DF) diet is also advisable. As mentioned before, wheat and dairy are very recent additions to the human diet. Our ancestors were hunter-gatherers; they did not eat wheat or dairy. Over a long period of time, they became genetically programmed to the hunter-gatherer diet.

Today we still have hunter-gatherer genes and have not yet adapted to the new, more recently introduced foods. We have caveman genes; we should eat caveman food.

Throughout this chapter, gluten has been discussed in the context of CD, yet there has been no discussion about what gluten actually is.

Gluten is a protein found in grains such as wheat, rye, barley, and oats.

The word gluten comes from the Latin *gluten* meaning 'glue'; this may make you consider whether you really want to eat it. It is a composite protein made up of two main proteins, gliadins and glutenins. Gliadin is the water-soluble component while glutenin is not. They are both relatively resistant to digestion even in a healthy gut (obviously if there are digestive problems then there can be an even greater issue). Humans have only one stomach and have difficulty digesting the protein unlike animals such as cows, sheep, and goats, that have multiple stomachs and can digest gluten. Even though they are proteins, they are not completely digested to the individual amino acids but are digested to shorter peptide chains. It is these shorter peptides that may cause the damage, with the main culprit being the gliadin protein, although other peptides may also cause problems.

When the partially digested peptide from gliadin reaches the intestine, the immune system reacts to it as if it were a foreign invader. This is possibly another example of molecular mimicry. *Tissue transglutaminase* modifies the gliadin peptide, and the immune system attacks this enzyme and damages the intestinal cells as collateral damage.

There have been articles on the internet saying that the rise of CD is due to the modern wheat being higher in gluten. This is not correct. The hallmark study by Kasarda (2013) showed no increase in gluten content in wheat since the beginning of the 20th century. However, the per capita consumption of wheat has increased.

de Lorgeril and Salen (2014) stated that *"Coeliac-triggering gluten proteins are indeed expressed to higher levels in modern cereals while non-triggering proteins are expressed less."*

Could it be that the actual level of gluten in wheat hasn't increased but the dangerous triggers are expressed more? This question was answered by van den Broeck et al. (2010) who looked at the wheat protein diversity. The researchers looked at two gluten epitomes, glia-α9 and glia-α20 in 36 modern European wheat varieties and 50 wheat varieties that were grown up to a century ago. The glia-α9 is the major (immunodominant) epitome that is recognised in most CD patients. The glia-α20, which doesn't seem to be reactive, was included as a technical reference. The study concluded that the level of glia-α9 was higher in modern wheat and the levels of glia-α20 were lower. The amount of gluten in the wheat isn't the problem, but the reactive fraction is becoming more prominent.

Why is it so hard to come off wheat/gluten?

The narrative of dieticians and doctors that unless you have CD, there is no need to come off gluten, is a consistent one, leading to many patients believing this to be true. Another reason is one not often spoken of, gluten can be addictive. Huebner, Lieberman, Rubino, and Wall (1984) demonstrated that gluten has been shown to break down to peptides that have opioid activity which can affect opioid receptors in the brain. These isolated opioid peptides were tested on rat's brains. The most active peptides were from the gliadin fraction of the gluten complex. Pruimboom and de Punder (2015) showed that gluten can be degraded into morphine-like substances called gluten exorphins. They discuss the interesting concept that the opioid effects of the gluten can "mask" its own toxicity.

The big question is, do these gluten exorphins get absorbed through the gut? A leaky gut does contribute. But can they cross the BBB? Ul Haq, (2020) showed that gluten exorphins do cross the BBB. Liu and Udenigwe (2019) concurred.

So, if gluten can produce opioids, then stopping gluten may produce withdrawal symptoms akin to drug withdrawal. Is this one reason it is hard to stop gluten? Some people do complain of symptoms when they try to stop eating gluten. Experiencing symptoms such as pain, tiredness, depression, weakness, anger and "brain fog" can drive the person back to eating that food again. In one way it does make sense as we know that opioid peptides are produced after the partial digestion of gluten. These peptides have been found in the brains in an animal model (Bressan & Kramer, 2016). Coming off opioids produces "withdrawal" symptoms. There are many anecdotal reports but unfortunately there are no peer reviewed studies.

The fascinating paper published in 2016 by Bressan and Kramer summarises much of what I have said above. The authors look at the effect wheat/gluten has, not just on the gut, but on the brain as well. In the earlier part of this chapter, I listed the psychiatric symptoms of depression and schizophrenia, which can be related to CD. An interesting statistic is that the rate of schizophrenia admissions to hospital declined during World War 2 in proportion to wheat shortages.

However, in the USA, during this same period, admission to hospital for schizophrenia rose, as there was no shortage of wheat in the USA, in fact, consumption rose. There could be many reasons for this,

WW2 being one of them, but the reference focused on wheat consumption. Gluten does resemble some brain substances so here again is a possibility of molecular mimicry. Above, I mentioned that there is a cross reaction with gluten antibodies and Purkinje cells and their relationship to "gluten ataxia." Gliadin antibodies are also similar to an enzyme that produces gamma amino butyric acid (GABA) which is an inhibiting neurotransmitter. This would cause issues with anxiety and depression. Gluten antibodies have been shown to be elevated much more often in patients with schizophrenia and autism than in the general population.

This could also answer another question. There is a well-established relationship between immigrant status and schizophrenia. Why? Certainly, when moving from poorer countries such as Africa to Europe the diet changes. The new immigrants receive a massive exposure to wheat (and therefore gluten) products which they have never experienced before. A gluten free and casein free diet has been shown to benefit patients with schizophrenia as well as children with autism.

Another question: Does gluten affect people who do not have CD? Bernardo, Garrote, Fernández-Salazar, Riestra, and Arranz (2007) showed that even in non-coeliac people, gluten can trigger some action in the gut, based on an interleukin 15 (Il 15) response.

Gut microbes also seem to play a part. They can

partly determine if (and when) CD gene carriers develop CD. What this can mean is that antibiotics in early life may predispose to CD in susceptible babies. I commented earlier that antibiotics are lifesaving but unfortunately are given on many occasions for trivial reasons. The maturation of the immune system is co-driven by the gut microbiota. The microbiota matures in the first twelve months of life, so inappropriate foods such as gluten should not be introduced during this time.

Another topic discussed in the Bressan and Kramer paper is the ability of gliadin proteins to cross the BBB. Although the experiment was done in rats, radioactive - labelled gluten was fed to rats and was later found in the brain as exorphins. Bressan and Kramer also discuss zonulin, which is a protein made by the gut. Zonulin controls the tight junction between the intestinal cells which can lead to LGS. Zonulin is released in response to pathogenic bacteria, as well as gliadin. Zonulin can also weaken the junctions in the BBB, allowing gliadin exorphins and other molecules to enter the brain. Not good! There may not only be a "leaky gut" but also a "leaky brain."

Inflammatory bowel disease (IBD)

"Thou shouldst eat to live; not live to eat."
Socrates (469 BC - 399 BC)

Irritable bowel syndrome (IBS) is sometimes referred to as irritable bowel disease (IBD), and this can be confusing. In this book, irritable bowel syndrome is IBS and inflammatory bowel disease is IBD.

IBD mainly refers to two diseases of unknown origin: ulcerative colitis (UC) and Crohn's disease (CrD). There are other forms of IBD, but this discussion will focus on the two most common ones. They are, as the name suggests, inflammatory diseases of the bowel. Although they are similar in some ways, they are essentially two very different diseases. I will try to explain the differences. While at times they may be difficult to differentiate, the aim of the following discussion is to explain the differences as clearly as possible.

As the treatment for any form of IBD including UC and CrD can be similar, it is not strictly necessary to differentiate between them. However, most patients do present after being investigated and having a diagnosis made.

Ulcerative colitis

UC is a disease where inflammation develops in the colon and produces ulcers. The disease mainly affects the colon, nearly always in the rectum and then spreads upwards and then stops abruptly. Rarely, the terminal ileum may be affected. In 25% of cases the disease is limited to the rectum only.

UC can come on any age but develops mainly in the 15 to 30 age group. It affects men and women equally and there may be some hereditary features, as it runs in some families.

Symptoms include diarrhoea, often with blood and pus, rectal bleeding, rectal pain, abdominal pain, weight loss, fever, and fatigue.

Crohn's disease

CrD also involves the bowel, mainly the colon, although it can develop anywhere from mouth to anus. It affects the:

- caecum and ileum in 40% of patients,
- small intestine only, in 30% of patients, and
- colon only, in 25% of patients.

The remaining 5% of sufferers develop CrD in mouth, tongue, oesophagus, stomach, or duodenum.

CrD is characterised by "skip lesions". There are areas of involvement where granulomatous inflammatory process is seen, with areas of normal bowel in between. In essence, lengths of bowel are "skipped" by the disease process. The other major difference is that in CrD, the pathological process involves all layers of the bowel, while UC mainly affects the superficial mucosa.

Symptoms include:

- diarrhoea, bloody diarrhoea is more typical of UC than CrD,
- abdominal pain, and
- inflammation with fever, malaise, nausea,

vomiting, sweats, and arthralgia.

IBD occurs in approximately 70-150 per 100,000 individuals, is four times more common amongst the white races, and is a disease of industrialised nations.

Dr Peter Baratosy MBBS FACNEM

Causes of IBD

Conventionally, the cause of IBD is listed as "not known". UC is considered to be an autoimmune disease, while CrD is thought to develop as collateral damage as a result of the immune system attacking a harmless virus, bacteria, or food in the gut.

The highest incidences of IBD are in North America, Northern Europe, and other developed countries. It is quite rare in developing countries.

It is also well known that the incidence of IBD has been increasing in the last 50-60 years. IBD is not only increasing in incidence but is also appearing in areas where it had never been before. This means that there must be some environmental factor. It cannot just be genetic.

These diseases were unknown in India prior to 1964 when the first case of UC was reported. CrD was considered almost non-existent until 1986 (Desai & Gupte, 2005).

A study in Sweden (Persson, Ahlbom, & Hellers,1992) showed an increase in incidence of IBD associated with the consumption of "fast foods." This was confirmed by Han, Anderson, Viennois, and Merlin (2020).

Reif et al. (1997) implicated a high sugar intake in the development of IBD, although this finding is not consistent and there are possibly other factors involved. The type of dietary carbohydrate seems to be more important in determining risk of IBD than the total intake of carbohydrate. Khademi, Milajerdi, Larijani, and Esmaillzadeh (2021) showed as did Reif et al. that there is increased risk associated with high sugar intake. Racine et al. (2016) found a positive association between "high sugar and soft drinks" pattern and UC risk but only in participants with a low vegetable intake.

Sugar intake is not healthy anyway!

Other factors implicated include sanitation, and drugs such as antibiotics and NSAIDs.

Before improvement of sanitation, many of the population were infected with intestinal worms, such as roundworms and hookworms. These worms have a blunting effect on gut immunity. As soon as sanitation improved, these worms disappeared from people's intestinal systems and soon after, IBD began to increase. This does not mean that improved sanitation is bad, however, it can have negative effects in some people (Desai & Gupte, 2005).

Some researchers say that worms can be a part of the normal microbiome. Ruyssers et al. (2008) showed that worms can be used to treat intestinal inflammation.

Summers, Elliott, Urban, Thompson, and Weinstock (2005) demonstrated the benefits of using worms, specifically the whipworm (*Trichuris suis*) in CrD. In a separate study carried out in the same year, the same group of researchers found that the worms can also be used in treating UC (Summers, Elliott, Urban, Thompson, & Weinstock, 2005).

Why do some with worms have problems and others not? There are many factors. A starving third world inhabitant with heavy infestation of worms may not get the benefits because they are malnourished and their whole immune system is probably very low, which is part of the problem. A relative healthy westerner with UC may benefit from worms. Perhaps it is due to balance. A good bacterial microbiome can keep the worms in check. The "hygiene hypothesis" which states that cleanliness is good but too clean is not good, may be relevant here. Our immune system needs things to fight against. If there is no external threat to fight, then the immune system fights the only thing left to fight: itself. The result is autoimmunity.

Antibiotics can cause a non-specific colitis which is neither UC nor CrD.

Conventionally, antibiotics are used to treat IBD when there is infection. Also, there is evidence that intestinal flora plays a pathogenic role in IBD, therefore when antibiotics are used to get rid of these pathogens an improvement in symptoms and induced remission has been shown to occur (Guslandi, 2005; Isaacs & Sartor, 2004). The antibiotic showing the most promise is rifaximin, mainly because it is largely a non-absorbable antibiotic, and therefore has fewer systemic effects (Gionchetti, Rizzello, Morselli, Romagnoli, & Campieri, 2005).

What about causation? Antibiotics can alter the microbiological flora of the gut and promote the over-growth of toxic bacteria. Can antibiotics given at an earlier stage alter gut flora to induce IBD? Card, Logan, Rodrigues, and Wheeler (2004) studied 587 patients with CrD and 1,460 controls. Antibiotic use 2-5 years pre-diagnosis occurred in 71% of patients with CrD and only 58% of controls, which means that there is an association between antibiotic use and CrD. Nguyen et al. (2020) also confirmed a link between antibiotic use and IBD.

As mentioned earlier the use of antibiotics is quite high as they are used indiscriminately for all sorts of trivial infections.

NSAIDs are drugs that do have a very irritating effect on the gut lining and can cause a non-specific colitis with subsequent complications such as ulcers, bleeding, perforation, and strictures. There is no evidence that NSAIDs can cause UC or CrD, but they can trigger exacerbations of UC and CrD (Thiéfin &

Beaugerie, 2005).

Short term use of NSAIDs appears to be safe, and the selective COX-2 inhibitors are safer. However, long term use should be avoided, especially in those with active inflammation (Hijos-Mallada, Sostres, & Gomollón, 2022).

Treatment of IBD

Other than conventional treatment, which will not be discussed here, there are alternatives. However, I must point out that in very acute, severe cases, the conventional treatment may be needed.

Unfortunately, you may not be informed about the alternative treatments. The following section will provide information that may be helpful. These may be used concurrently with conventional treatment.

Many of the standard medical web sites say there is no special diet for IBD.

They confirm, however, that people with IBD need a nutritious diet and they are correct about that as many who suffer IBD are often malnourished because their gut is not working properly.

Conventional wisdom focuses on providing nutrients to prevent and/or reverse malnutrition and to prevent weight loss.

Diet

As mentioned, many times, there are some foods that humans should not be eating. While some people can tolerate grains and dairy, many cannot. There is no specific evidence that grains and dairy cause IBD but Weaver and Herfarth (2021) provided evidence that eliminating gluten from the diet may help people with IBD. However, there is minimal evidence for the benefit of eliminating dairy. As mentioned earlier, there is no need to wait for scientific evidence. If dairy makes you feel unwell, and/or makes your condition worse, how you feel is enough evidence that limiting dairy foods from your diet is worth trying.

Giving nutrition intravenously (total parenteral nutrition, TPN) can be very useful. Seo, Okada, Yao, Furukawa, and Matake (1999) studied patients with acute attacks of IBD who were given steroids and either TPN or the usual hospital diet. In patients with UC there was no difference, but patients with CrD showed great improvement with the TPN.

The above studies show that what goes in through the mouth influences the gastrointestinal system. Many of my patients were told by their regular health care providers that diet was not important in IBD. However, evidence about the benefits of diet in treating IBD is now appearing in peer-reviewed journals. As recently as 2018, Reddavide et al. wrote, *"Among the environmental factors associated with IBD, diet plays an important role in modulating the gut microbiome, and, consequently, it could have a therapeutic impact on the disease course."*

Fish oil

Fish oil, specifically omega 3 fatty acids, have anti-inflammatory actions and therefore, logically would be useful in IBD. Siguel and Lerman (1996) showed that patients with chronic intestinal disorders are deficient in essential fatty acids (EFA) due to malabsorption and nutritional losses through diarrhoea. Marton, Goulart, Carvalho, and Barbalho (2019) showed that omega 3 can reduce intestinal inflammation and, as well, can reduce the risk of developing IBD. Belluzzi et al. (1996) and Tsujikawa et al. (2000) confirmed that fish oil supplementation can reduce relapse rates in CrD. Aslan and Triadafilopoulos in 1992 demonstrated that fish oil produced improvement in mild to moderate cases of UC.

In a study of UC patients by Seidner et al. (2005) an oral supplement which contained fish oil, fructooligosaccharides (FOS), gum arabic, vitamin E, vitamin C and selenium was compared with a placebo. The supplemented group had a much greater clinical response as well as a reduced requirement for steroid medication.

Glutamine

Glutamine has already been discussed in the context of LGS. To review, glutamine is an amino acid that is the preferred nutrition for intestinal cells. If it is good for non-serious disease, is it also good for serious disease? The answer is "yes."

Fujita and Sakurai (1995) showed that a glutamine-enriched diet may be therapeutic for patients with IBD, although this conclusion was based on a guinea pig model.

Kanauchi et al. (2003) found that germinated barley foodstuff (GBF) which is glutamine rich was used in patients with UC and it was highly beneficial. GBF is not only rich in glutamine but also acts as a prebiotic that increases butyrate production by stimulating protective gut bacteria. Although, GBF, which is made from barley, may contain gluten.

Glutamine has also been used in unspecified critical illness. Kelly and Wischmeyer (2003) discussed that glutamine supplementation has been used for many years and has shown benefit with respect to mortality, length of hospital stays and infectious morbidity. They also made the comment that no evidence of harm has been observed.

Dr Peter Baratosy MBBS FACNEM

Probiotics

Probiotics have already been discussed, but in the following discussion the focus will be specifically on probiotic use in IBD. It is well known and accepted that probiotics are beneficial for general gut problems and now there is mounting evidence that they are also useful in the treatment of more serious diseases such as IBD.

Now that it is known that bacteria (especially pathogenic bacteria) can initiate and perpetuate IBD, it makes sense that "good" bacteria could possibly treat and prevent relapses.

Bibilone et al. (2005) studied a specific commercial probiotic formula called VSL#3®, (*https://vsl3.com*). This particular blend of probiotics was shown to induce remission in active UC. See also Ciorba (2012) and appendix 3.

Unfortunately, the evidence is not so good for CrD. The results of a study by Prantera, Scribano, Falasco, Andreoli, and Luzi (2002) showed there was no benefit when the probiotic *Lactobacillus GG was used* in CrD.

It is highly likely that many with CrD probably have been on antibiotics at some stage of their illness. So, despite the above negative result, using probiotics in

CrD is still worth the effort. As mentioned earlier not all probiotics are the same and as previously suggested, if you do use a probiotic formula, it is good to use different brands to get an increasing variety of bacteria strains from different manufacturers. Dosage should be based on severity. Large doses, three to four times the recommended dose, should be used in acute illness, and the recommended dose for maintenance.

One probiotic worth considering is *Saccharomyces boulardii*. This is not a bacterial probiotic but a non-pathogenic fungus. This probiotic has been shown to be of benefit in both UC (Guslandi, Giollo, & Testoni, 2003) and CrD (Guslandi, Mezzi, Sorghi, & Testoni, 2000).

EcN has also been mentioned previously. This is another probiotic that has been shown to help with CrD and UC. Although the table in Ciorba's (2012) paper did not refer to EcN in relation to CrD, there may be some benefit. A pilot study (Malchow, 1997) looked at CrD and EcN and showed benefit for maintaining remission, although the study concluded with the usual caveat; *"more data are necessary to prove the benefit."*

EcN has been shown to be beneficial in UC. According to Kruis et al. (2004) EcN is as effective at maintaining remission in UC as mesalazine, a conventionally used drug in UC.

Herbs

I have discussed some herbs already. These can be used in IBD as well as in other gastrointestinal problems.

One of the main herbs used in gastrointestinal disease is SEB, which I have already stated is a very soothing herb. It makes sense to use a soothing herb on an inflamed gastrointestinal lining.

Langmead et al. (2002) showed that SEB had an antioxidant effect on gut mucosa and could be a useful herb in IBD. Other herbs assessed in this study, with positive effects, include fenugreek, devil's claw, tormentil and wei tong ning (a traditional Chinese medicine).

Another soothing, healing, anti-inflammatory herb is aloe vera. Langmead et al. (2004) found that oral aloe vera gel produced clinical improvement in active UC after four weeks of use.

Another useful herb is curcumin, an active extract of turmeric (*Curcuma longa*), one of the components of curry. It is an exceptionally useful herb, and its main action is as an anti-inflammatory. Hence its use in inflammatory diseases of the gut. Fallahi et al. (2021) demonstrated that curcumin can reduce inflammation in IBD. NSAIDs are anti-inflammatory but have a side effect of gut irritation, to the point of bleeding. Curcumin is a natural anti-inflammatory that reduces gut inflammation rather than causing it.

Dr Peter Baratosy MBBS FACNEM

CBD oil

The endocannabinoid system (ECS) and the use of CBD oil in treating diseases has been discussed previously. IBD is another category of diseases that responds to CBD oil. CBD oil can be used in the treatment of CrD and UC because it reduces inflammation and works through other mechanisms as well (Esposito et al., 2013; Di Carlo & Izzo, 2003; Schicho & Storr, 2014).

In a story from the Australian Broadcasting Commission (ABC) 7.30 report, 7 March 2018, a father was treating his sick daughters with cannabis. Both daughters had severe CrD and they were on many pharmaceutical medications and were not doing well: they were dying. The father took matters into his own hands and started treating them with cannabis leaf smoothies. He was using the leaf and stem only which does not contain much, if any, of the psychoactive THC: the leaf contains mainly cannabidiol (CBD). Within weeks they were putting on weight and becoming much better. He was raided by the police and charged with cultivation and possession of cannabis. Eventually he was put on a good behaviour bond rather than jailed!

Professor Iain McGregor, professor of Psychopharmacy at the Lambert Initiative for

Cannabinoid Therapeutics at Sydney University explained, "*Juicing cannabis is much different than smoking it.*" He continued, "*In many ways, juicing is a positive thing to do because you don't get nearly as much of the intoxicating element, which is THC [tetrahyrdocannabinol] and you get another component of cannabinoid, which is THCA [tetrahydocannabinolic acid], which has very strong anti-inflammatory properties in the gut.*" (ABC News Updated 8 Mar 2018)

Heating cannabis by burning, smoking, cooking, etc., converts tetrahydrocannabinolic acid (THCA) which is not psychoactive to tetrahydrocannabinol (THC) which is psychoactive. So, eating cannabis as a salad or as a smoothie does not have psychoactive effects.

PEA, discussed earlier, has been shown to reduce inflammation and pain in CrD and UC (Sałaga, Sobczak, & Fichna, 2014; Esposito et al., 2014; Borrelli et al., 2015; Sarnelli et al., 2016).

Dr Peter Baratosy MBBS FACNEM

Low dose naltrexone (LDN)

Naltrexone is a conventional drug used in emergency medicine to revive patients who have overdosed on narcotics. Its mode of action is to block the opioid receptors. In emergency medicine the dose can be as high as 100-150 mgs. When using LDN the dose is as low as 4.5 mgs.

The main protocol used is 1.5 mgs for the first 4 weeks, then increase to 3 mgs for the next 4 weeks then 4.5 mgs thereafter.

How does it work?

The simple idea of its mode of action is that the naltrexone temporarily blocks the endorphin (opioid) receptors. The body, in response, produces a rebound increase in endorphins. Once the LDN has worn off, usually after a few hours, the higher levels of endorphins have a positive effect on the body, producing pain relief and anti-inflammation. Donahue, McLaughlin, and Zagon (2011) have shown that the action of LDN is more complex than indicated above and it has been demonstrated to target the opioid growth factor (OGF) and the OGF Receptor (OGFr) axis.

LDN has been used in many conditions, especially MS, fibromyalgia, chronic fatigue syndrome, chronic pain, Hashimoto's thyroiditis and IBD. It is also very useful in situations where you don't know what else to do.

There is evidence that LDN is effective (Younger, Parkitny, & McLain, 2014; Patten, Schultz, & Berlau, 2018; Metyas, Chen, Yeter, Solyman, & Arkfeld, 2018).

I have treated patients with MS, UC, and chronic fatigue with LDN with positive results.

Summary

"A Short History of Medicine

2000BC- Here, eat this root.

1000BC- That root is heathen, say this prayer.

1850AD- That prayer is superstition, drink this potion.

1920 AD- That potion is snake oil, swallow this pill.

1945AD- That pill is ineffective, take this penicillin.

1955 AD- Oops...bugs mutated, take this tetracycline.

1960 – 1999 AD- Thirty-nine more oops – take this more powerful antibiotic.

2000AD- That antibiotic is artificial. Here, eat this root."

Author Unknown

Gastrointestinal problems are very common in today's western society. We are facing an epidemic of chronic disease in which gut problems are the rule, not the exception. During my years of clinical practice, I learned that if the gut issues are not addressed, then the response will be sub optimal in whatever chronic condition you are treating. I also learned that in a complicated case, the best place to start is to treat the gut first. It is always surprising how much improvement there is!

Standard treatments consist mainly of "anti" treatments: anti-acid, anti-pain, anti-bloating, anti-diarrhoea, anti-constipation, and the rest.

While these treatments may give temporary symptomatic relief they do not get to the root of the problem.

On the contrary, they may lead to extra long-term problems. What I have attempted in this book is to outline a simple, natural approach to gastrointestinal problems, with an emphasis on trying to deal with the root problem. The greatest root problem is the western diet.

Our species has not evolved fast enough to keep up with this un-natural eating pattern.

Foods such as grains, dairy and sugar are not meant to be eaten by humans, or perhaps only occasionally, and in small amounts.

The western diet is not conducive to well-being.

If the diet is improved, then so will the health of the nation.

Unfortunately, one of the main barriers to this change in diet is the resistance by the food manufacturers themselves. Food, and what we are told is good for us, has become an economic and political issue.

The answer to the health problems is simple. However, the necessary changes would be difficult to achieve, primarily because the wheat, sugar and dairy farmers and manufacturers would be fighting tooth and nail to resist any change.

Our genes are still caveman/woman. We, therefore, should eat like caveman/woman, or as close to how they ate as possible. Despite resistance from business and politicians, everyone has the capacity to make a decision that will enhance their wellbeing, and possibly increase life expectancy. My hope is that this book will help you to do that.

In summary, a simple and natural approach can prevent many of the problems that have developed in today's society.

The KISS Principle: Keep it Simple, Stupid.

Appendix 1

BRISTOL STOOL CHART

	Type 1	Separate hard lumps	Very constipated
	Type 2	Lumpy and sausage like	Slightly constipated
	Type 3	A sausage shape with cracks in the surface	Normal
	Type 4	Like a smooth, soft sausage or snake	Normal
	Type 5	Soft blobs with clear-cut edges	Lacking fibre
	Type 6	Mushy consistency with ragged edges	Inflammation
	Type 7	Liquid consistency with no solid pieces	Inflammation

Appendix 2

Fungus Related Disease Questionnaire-7 (FRDQ-7).

SCORE: 0 = none

1 = occasional or mild

2 = frequent or moderately severe

3 = severe or disabling or Yes

1. Have you, at any time in your life, taken broad spectrum antibiotics? 0 or 3

2. Have you taken tetracycline or other broad-spectrum antibiotics for one month or longer? 0 or 3

3. Are your symptoms worse on damp, muggy days or in mouldy places? 0 or 3

4. Do you crave sugar? 0 or 3

5. Do you have a feeling of being "drained?" 0, 1, 2 or 3

6. WOMEN: Are you bothered with vaginal burning, itching or discharge? 0, 1, 2 or 3

MEN: Do you have burning, itching or discharge from the penis? 0, 1, 2 or 3

7. Are you bothered by burning, itching, or tearing of your eyes? 0, 1, 2 or 3

TOTAL SCORE FOR FRDQ-7:

Score   0-3   =   FRD unlikely

Score   4-9   =   FRD probable

Score 10-21 =   FRD almost certain

(© Marjorie Crandall, Ph.D)

Appendix 3

<u>Explanation</u> – Effectiveness:

A – Some positive well conducted studies.

B – Some positive controlled studies but some negative studies or inadequate work to establish the certainty.

C – Some positive studies but clearly inadequate amount of work to establish certainty.

<u>Abbreviations:</u> CDAD – Clostridium difficile associated diarrhoea

AAD   Antibiotic associated diarrhoea

IBS   irritable bowel syndrome

UC   ulcerative colitis

CD   Crohn's disease

B   Bifidobacterium

L   Lactobacillus

S   Saccharomyces

NS   no explanation – assume Not Specified

B/C   no explanation – assume somewhere between B and C.

Note – the number after the species refers to the strain.

Bacterial Species	Clinical Condition	Effectiveness
B. lactis DN-1173 010, *L. bulgaricus* *L. lactis,* *Strep. thermophilus*	IBS	C
B. infantis 35624	IBS	B
L. reuteri protectis *SD2112(ATCC*	Infectious diarrhoea treatment	A
55730 or DSM 17928	IBS	C
L. acidophillus DL1285 and *L. casei LBC80R*	AAD prevention CDAD prevention	NS
L. rhamnosus GG	AAD prevention	A
	Infectious diarrhoea treatment	A
	Infectious diarrhoea prevention	B
	CDAD prevention	B/C
	CDAD prevention of recurrence	B/C
	Crohn's disease	C
	IBS	B/C
L. casei DN 114001	AAD	A
	Infectious diarrhoea prevention	

CDAD prevention

S. boulardii	AAD prevention	A
	Infectious diarrhoea treatment	A
	Infectious diarrhoea prevention	B
	CDAD prevention	B/C
	CDAD prevention of recurrence	B/C
	Crohn's disease	C

E. coli Nissle 1917	UC induction	B
	UC maintenance	A

VSL#3 ®	IBS	B/C
Mixture various species	UC induction	B
	UC maintenance	A
	Pouchitis	
	Prevention and	
	maintaining remission.	A

Adapted from Ciorba, (2012).

References

Aagaard, K., Ma, J., Antony, K., Ganu, R., Petrosino, J. & Versalovic, J. (2014). The placenta harbors a unique microbiome. *Sci Transl Med, 6*(237):237ra65. doi: 10.1126/scitranslmed.3008599

Achamrah, N., Déchelotte, P. & Coëffier, M. (2017). Glutamine and the regulation of intestinal permeability: from bench to bedside. *Curr Opin Clin Nutr Metab Care, 20*(1), 86-91. doi: 10.1097/MCO.0000000000000339

Agranoff, B. & Goldberg, D. (1974). Diet and the geographical distribution of multiple sclerosis. *Lancet, 2*(7888), 1061-6. doi: 10.1016/s0140-6736(74)92163-1

Agrawal, A., Nelson, E., Littlefield, A., Bucholz, K., Degenhardt, L., Henders, A., … Lynskey, M. (2012). Cannabinoid receptor genotype moderation of the effects of childhood physical abuse on anhedonia and depression. *Arch Gen Psychiatry, 69*(7), 732-40. doi: 10.1001/archgenpsychiatry.2011.2273

Ahn, K., Johnson, D. & Cravatt, B. (2009). Fatty acid amide hydrolase as a potential therapeutic target for the treatment of pain and CNS disorders. *Expert Opin Drug Discov, 4*(7), 763-784. doi:

10.1517/17460440903018857

Al-Bakri, A., Othman, G. & Afifi, F. (2010). Determination of the antibiofilm, antiadhesive, and anti-MRSA activities of seven Salvia species. *Pharmacogn Mag, 6*(24), 264-70. doi: 10.4103/0973-1296.71786

Aldoori, W., Giovannucci, E., Rimm, E., Wing, A., Trichopoulos, D. & Willett, W. (1994). A prospective study of diet and the risk of symptomatic diverticular disease in men. *Am J Clin Nutr, 60*(5), 757-64. doi: 10.1093/ajcn/60.5.757

Aleman, R., Moncada, M. & Aryana, K. (2023). Leaky gut and the ingredients that help treat it: A review. *Molecules, 28*(2), 619. doi: 10.3390/molecules28020619

Allen, S., Okoko, B., Martinez, E., Gregorio, G. & Dans, LF. (2004). Probiotics for treating infectious diarrhoea. *Cochrane Database Syst Rev,* (2), CD003048. doi: 10.1002/14651858.CD003048.pub2

Alvarez-Arellano, L., & Maldonado-Bernal, C. (2014). Helicobacter pylori and neurological diseases: Married by the laws of inflammation. World J Gastrointest Pathophysiol. 2014 Nov 15;5(4):400-4. doi: 10.4291/wjgp.v5.i4.400

Amedei, A., Codolo, G., Del Prete, G., de Bernard, M.

& D'Elios, M. (2010). The effect of Helicobacter pylori on asthma and allergy. *J Asthma Allergy, 3*, 139-47. doi: 10.2147/JAA.S8971

Andersen, B., Johansen, P. & Abrahamsen, B. (2016). Proton pump inhibitors and osteoporosis. *Curr Opin Rheumatol, 28*(4), 420-5. doi: 10.1097/BOR.0000000000000291

Andersen, B., Scheel, J., Rune, S. & Worning, H. (1982). Exocrine pancreatic function in patients with dyspepsia. *Hepatogastroenterology, 29*(1),35-7.

Andersen, J., Bundgaard, L., Elbrønd, H., Laurberg, S., Walker, L & Støvring J; Danish Surgical Society. (2012). Danish national guidelines for treatment of diverticular disease. *Dan Med J, 59*(5), C4453

Arce, D., Ermocilla, C., & Costa, H. (2002). Evaluation of constipation. *Am Fam Physician, 65*(11), 2283-90.

Arnold, I., Dehzad, N., Reuter, S., Martin, H., Becher, B., Taube, C. & Müller, A. (2011). Helicobacter pylori infection prevents allergic asthma in mouse models through the induction of regulatory T cells. *J Clin Invest, 121*(8), 3088-93. doi: 10.1172/JCI45041

Aslan, A. & Triadafilopoulos, G. (1992). Fish oil fatty acid supplementation in active ulcerative colitis: a double-blind, placebo-controlled, crossover study. *Am J Gastroenterol, 87*(4), 432-7

Aune, D., Sen, A., Leitzmann, M., Tonstad, S., Norat, T. & Vatten, L. (2017). Tobacco smoking and the risk of diverticular disease - a systematic review and meta-analysis of prospective studies. *Colorectal Dis, 19*(7), 621-633. doi: 10.1111/codi.13748

Awasthi, S., Peto, R., Read, S., Richards, S., Pande, V., Bundy, D.; DEVTA (Deworming and Enhanced Vitamin A) team. (2013). Population deworming every 6 months with albendazole in 1 million pre-school children in North India: DEVTA, a cluster-randomised trial. *Lancet, 381*(9876), 1478-86. doi: 10.1016/S0140-6736(12)62126-6

Bajaj, J., Heuman, D., Hylemon, P., Sanyal, A., Puri, P., Sterling, R., ... Gillevet, P. (2014). Randomised clinical trial: Lactobacillus GG modulates gut microbiome, metabolome and endotoxemia in patients with cirrhosis. *Aliment Pharmacol Ther, 39*(10), 1113-25. doi: 10.1111/apt.12695

Balaghi, M. & Wagner, C. (1995). Folate deficiency inhibits pancreatic amylase secretion in rats. *Am J Clin Nutr, 61*(1), 90-6. doi: 10.1093/ajcn/61.1.90

Basheer, A., Mookkappan, S., Shanmugham, V. & Natarajan, N. (2014). Hepatitis-B associated acute transverse myelitis mimicking syringomyelia. *J Case Reports, 4*, 77-81. doi: 10.17659/01.2014.0019

Bavishi, C. & Dupont, H. (2011). Systematic review:

the use of proton pump inhibitors and increased susceptibility to enteric infection. *Aliment Pharmacol Ther, 34*(11-12), 1269-81. doi: 10.1111/j.1365-2036.2011.04874.x

Belluzzi, A., Brignola, C., Campieri, M., Pera, A., Boschi, S. & Miglioli, M. (1996). Effect of an enteric-coated fish-oil preparation on relapses in Crohn's disease. *N Engl J Med, 334*(24), 1557-60. doi: 10.1056/NEJM199606133342401

Bennett, D., Baird, C., Chan, K., Crookes, P., Bremner, C., Gottlieb, M. & Naritoku, W. (1997). Zinc toxicity following massive coin ingestion. *Am J Forensic Med Pathol, 18*(2),148-53. doi: 10.1097/00000433-199706000-00008

Bernardo, D., Garrote, J., Fernández-Salazar, L., Riestra, S. & Arranz, E. (2007). Is gliadin really safe for non-coeliac individuals? Production of interleukin 15 in biopsy culture from non-coeliac individuals challenged with gliadin peptides. *Gut, 56*(6), 889-90. doi: 10.1136/gut.2006.118265

Bibiloni, R., Fedorak, R., Tannock, G., Madsen, K., Gionchetti, P., Campieri, M., … Sartor, R. (2005). VSL#3 probiotic-mixture induces remission in patients with active ulcerative colitis. *Am J Gastroenterol, 100*(7), 1539-46. doi: 10.1111/j.1572-0241.2005.41794.x

Bjarnsholt, T., Alhede, M., Jensen, P., Nielsen, A., Johansen, H., Homøe, P., ... Kirketerp-Møller, K. (2015). Antibiofilm properties of acetic acid. *Adv Wound Care (New Rochelle), 4*(7), 363-372. doi: 10.1089/wound.2014.0554

Blaser, M., Chen, Y. & Reibman, J. (2008). Does Helicobacter pylori protect against asthma and allergy? *Gut. 2008, 57*(5), 561-7. doi: 10.1136/gut.2007.133462

Borrelli, F., Romano, B., Petrosino, S., Pagano, E., Capasso, R., Coppola, D., ... Izzo,A. (2015). Palmitoylethanolamide, a naturally occurring lipid, is an orally effective intestinal anti-inflammatory agent. *Br J Pharmacol, 172*(1), 142-58. doi: 10.1111/bph.12907

Brackman, G. & Coenye, T. (2015). Quorum sensing inhibitors as anti-biofilm agents. *Curr Pharm Des, 21*(1), 5-11. doi: 10.2174/1381612820666140905114627

Brechmann, T., Sperlbaum, A. & Schmiegel, W. (2017). Levothyroxine therapy and impaired clearance are the strongest contributors to small intestinal bacterial overgrowth: Results of a retrospective cohort study. *World J Gastroenterol, 23*(5), 842-852. doi: 10.3748/wjg.v23.i5.842

Bredenoord, A., Weusten, B., Sifrim, D., Timmer, R. & Smout, A. (2004). Aerophagia, gastric, and supragastric belching: a study using intraluminal electrical impedance monitoring. *Gut, 53*(11). 1561-5. doi: 10.1136/gut.2004.042945

Bredenoord, A., Weusten, B., Timmer, R. & Smout, A. (2006). Psychological factors affect the frequency of belching in patients with aerophagia. *Am J Gastroenterol, 101*(12), 2777-81. doi: 10.1111/j.1572-0241.2006.00917.x

Bressan, P. & Kramer, P. (2016). Bread and other edible agents of mental disease. *Front Hum Neurosci,10*, 130. doi: 10.3389/fnhum.2016.00130

Britton, E. & McLaughlin, J. (2013). Ageing and the gut. *Proc Nutr Soc, 72*(1),173-7. doi: 10.1017/S0029665112002807

Brown, L. (2000). Helicobacter pylori: epidemiology and routes of transmission. *Epidemiol Rev, 22*(2), 283-97. doi: 10.1093/oxfordjournals.epirev.a018040

Brown, P. (1976). The influence of smoking on pancreatic function in man. *Med J Aust, 2*(8), 290-3. doi: 10.5694/j.1326-5377.1976.tb130184.x

Bruckschen, E. & Horosiewicz, H. (1994). Chronische obstipation, vergleich von mikrobiologischer therapie und lactulose. *Munch med Wochenschr, 16*, 241-5.

Budzyński, J. & Kłopocka, M. (2014). Brain-gut axis in the pathogenesis of Helicobacter pylori infection.

World J Gastroenterol, 20(18), 5212-25. doi:
10.3748/wjg.v20.i18.5212

Bulka, C., Davis, M., Karagas, M., Ahsan, H. & Argos,
M. (2017). The unintended consequences of a gluten-
free diet. *Epidemiology, 28*(3), e24-e25. doi:
10.1097/EDE.0000000000000640

Bustos Fernández, L., Man, F. & Lasa, J. (2023).
Impact of Saccharomyces boulardii CNCM I-745 on
bacterial overgrowth and composition of intestinal
microbiota in IBS-D patients: results of a randomized
pilot study. *Dig Dis*, Jan 11. doi: 10.1159/000528954.
Epub ahead of print.

Cañizares, P., Gracia, I., Gómez, L., Martín de Argila,
C., de Rafael, L. & García, A. (2002). Optimization of
Allium sativum solvent extraction for the inhibition of
in vitro growth of Helicobacter pylori. *Biotechnol Prog,
18*(6), 1227-32. doi: 10.1021/bp025592z

Cao, Y., Strate, L., Keeley, B., Tam, I., Wu, K.,
Giovannucci, E., Chan, A. (2018). Meat intake and risk
of diverticulitis among men. *Gut, 67*(3), 466-472. doi:
10.1136/gutjnl-2016-313082

Card, T., Logan, R., Rodrigues, L. & Wheeler, J.
(2004). Antibiotic use and the development of Crohn's
disease. *Gut, 53*(2), 246-50. doi:
10.1136/gut.2003.025239

Chan, J., Carr, I. & Mayberry, J. (1997). The role of acupuncture in the treatment of irritable bowel syndrome: a pilot study. *Hepatogastroenterology, 44*(17), 1328-30.

Chander Roland, B., Mullin, G., Passi, M., Zheng, X., Salem, A., Yolken, R., & Pasricha P. (2017). A Prospective evaluation of ileocecal valve dysfunction and intestinal motility derangements in small intestinal bacterial overgrowth. *Dig Dis Sci, 62*(12), 3525-3535. doi: 10.1007/s10620-017-4726-4

Chao, G. & Zhang, S. (2014). Effectiveness of acupuncture to treat irritable bowel syndrome: a meta-analysis. *World J Gastroenterol, 20*(7), 1871-7. doi: 10.3748/wjg.v20.i7.1871

Chedid, V., Dhalla, S., Clarke, J., Roland, B., Dunbar, K., Koh, J., … Mullin, G. (2014). Herbal therapy is equivalent to rifaximin for the treatment of small intestinal bacterial overgrowth. *Glob Adv Health Med,3*(3), 16-24. doi: 10.7453/gahmj.2014.019

Christian, L., Galley, J., Hade, E., Schoppe-Sullivan, S., Kamp Dush, C. & Bailey, M. (2015). Gut microbiome composition is associated with temperament during early childhood. *Brain Behav Immun, 45*, 118-27. doi: 10.1016/j.bbi.2014.10.018

Ciorba, M. (2012). A gastroenterologist's guide to probiotics. *Clin Gastroenterol Hepatol, 10*(9), 960-8. doi: 10.1016/j.cgh.2012.03.024

Collinson, S., Deans, A., Padua-Zamora, A., Gregorio, G., Li, C., Dans, L. & Allen, S. (2020). Probiotics for treating acute infectious diarrhoea. *Cochrane Database Syst Rev, 12*(12), CD003048. doi: 10.1002/14651858.CD003048.pub4

Compare, D., Pica, L., Rocco, A., De Giorgi, F., Cuomo, R., Sarnelli, G., ... Nardone, G. (2011). Effects of long-term PPI treatment on producing bowel symptoms and SIBO. *Eur J Clin Invest, 41*(4):380-6. doi: 10.1111/j.1365-2362.2010.02419.x

Cryan, J. & Dinan, T. (2012). Mind-altering microorganisms: the impact of the gut microbiota on brain and behaviour. *Nat Rev Neurosci, 13*(10),701-12. doi: 10.1038/nrn3346

Cusick, M., Libbey, J., & Fujinami, R. (2012). Molecular mimicry as a mechanism of autoimmune disease. *Clin Rev Allergy Immunol, 42*(1), 102-11. doi: 10.1007/s12016-011-8294-7

Daher, S., Tahan, S., Solé, D., Naspitz, C., Da Silva Patrício, F., Neto, U. & De Morais, M. (2001). Cow's milk protein intolerance and chronic constipation in children. *Pediatr Allergy Immunol, 12*(6), 339-42. doi: 10.1034/j.1399-3038.2001.0o057.x de Goffau, M., Lager, S., Sovio, U., Gaccioli, F., Cook, E., Peacock, S., … Smith, G. (2019). Human placenta has no microbiome but can contain potential pathogens. *Nature, 572*(7769), 329-334. doi: 10.1038/s41586-019-1451-5

de Lorgeril, M & Salen, P. (2014). Gluten and wheat intolerance today: are modern wheat strains involved? *Int J Food Sci Nutr, 65*(5), 577-81. doi: 10.3109/09637486.2014.886185

Desai, H. & Gupte, P. (2005). Increasing incidence of Crohn's disease in India: is it related to improved sanitation? *Indian J Gastroenterol, 24*(1), 23-4.

D'Eufemia, P., Celli, M., Finocchiaro, R., Pacifico, L., Viozzi, L., Zaccagnini, M., … Giardini, O. (1996). Abnormal intestinal permeability in children with autism. *Acta Paediatr, 85*(9), 1076-9. doi: 10.1111/j.1651-2227.1996.tb14220.x

Di Carlo, G. & Izzo, A. (2003). Cannabinoids for gastrointestinal diseases: potential therapeutic applications. *Expert Opin Investig Drugs, 12*(1), 39-49. doi: 10.1517/13543784.12.1.39

Di Carlo, G. & Izzo, A. (2003). Cannabinoids for gastrointestinal diseases: potential therapeutic applications. *Expert Opin Investig Drugs, 12*(1):39-49. doi: 10.1517/13543784.12.1.39

Di Francesco, A., Falconi, A., Di Germanio, C., Micioni Di Bonaventura, M., Costa, A., Caramuta, S. ... D'Addario, C. (2015). Extravirgin olive oil up-regulates CB_1 tumor suppressor gene in human colon cancer cells and in rat colon via epigenetic mechanisms. *J Nutr Biochem, 26*(3), 250-8. doi: 10.1016/j.jnutbio.2014.10.013

di Tomaso, E., Beltramo, M. & Piomelli, D. (1996). Brain cannabinoids in chocolate. *Nature, 382*(6593), 677-8. doi: 10.1038/382677a0

Dobbs, R., Dobbs, S., Weller C, Charlett A, Bjarnason IT, Curry A, ... Williams J. (2008). Helicobacter hypothesis for idiopathic parkinsonism: before and beyond. *Helicobacter, 13*(5), 309-22. doi: 10.1111/j.1523-5378.2008.00622.x

Donahue, R, McLaughlin, P. & Zagon, I. (2011). Low-dose naltrexone targets the opioid growth factor-opioid growth factor receptor pathway to inhibit cell proliferation: mechanistic evidence from a tissue culture model. *Exp Biol Med (Maywood), 236*(9), 1036-50. doi: 10.1258/ebm.2011.011121

Droste, J., Wieringa, M., Weyler, J., Nelen, V., Vermeire, P. & Van Bever, H. (2000). Does the use of antibiotics in early childhood increase the risk of asthma and allergic disease? *Clin Exp Allergy, 30*(11), 1547-53. doi: 10.1046/j.1365-2222.2000.00939.x

Duggan, J. (2004). Coeliac disease: the great imitator. *Med J Aust, 180*(10), 524-6. doi: 10.5694/j.1326-5377.2004.tb06058.x

Dukowicz, A., Lacy, B. & Levine, G. (2007). Small intestinal bacterial overgrowth: a comprehensive review. *Gastroenterol Hepatol (N Y), 3*(2), 112-22

Dukowicz, A., Lacy, B. & Levine, G. (2007). Small intestinal bacterial overgrowth: a comprehensive review. *Gastroenterol Hepatol (N Y), 3*(2), 112-22

Dukowicz, A., Lacy, B. & Levine, G. (2007). Small intestinal bacterial overgrowth: comprehensive review. *Gastroenterol Hepatol (N Y), 3*(2), 112-22

Dutta, P., Mitra, U., Datta, A., Niyogi, S., Dutta, S., Manna, B., … Bhattacharya, S. (2000). Impact of zinc supplementation in malnourished children with acute watery diarrhoea. *J Trop Pediatr, 46*(5), 259-63. doi: 10.1093/tropej/46.5.259

Dutta, S., Procaccino, F. & Aamodt, R. (1998). Zinc metabolism in patients with exocrine pancreatic insufficiency. *J Am Coll Nutr, 17*(6), 556-63. doi: 10.1080/07315724.1998.10718803

Ebringer, A., Hughes, L., Rashid, T., & Wilson, C. (2005). Molecular Mimicry. In: Vohr, HW. (eds) Encyclopedic Reference of Immunotoxicology. Springer, Berlin, Heidelberg. https://doi.org/10.1007/3-

540-27806-0_1012

El-Hodhod, M., Nassar, M., Hetta, O. & Gomaa, S. (2005). Pancreatic size in protein energy malnutrition: a predictor of nutritional recovery. *Eur J Clin Nutr, 59*(4), 467-73. doi: 10.1038/sj.ejcn.1602053

El-Mowafy, S., Shaaban, M. & Abd El Galil, K. (2014). Sodium ascorbate as a quorum sensing inhibitor of Pseudomonas aeruginosa. *J Appl Microbiol, 117*(5):1388-99. doi: 10.1111/jam.12631

Elwyn, G., Taubert, M., Davies, S., Brown, G., Allison, M. & Phillips, C. (2007). Which test is best for Helicobacter pylori? A cost-effectiveness model using decision analysis. *Br J Gen Pract, 57*(538), 401-3.

Enders, G. (2015). *Gut*, Scribe Publications. ISBN: 9781771643764 Australia

Esplugues, J., Barrachina, M., Beltrán, B., Calatayud, S., Whittle, B. & Moncada, S. (1996). Inhibition of gastric acid secretion by stress: a protective reflex mediated by cerebral nitric oxide. *Proc Natl Acad Sci U S A, 93*(25),14839-44. doi: 10.1073/pnas.93.25.14839

Esposito, G., Capoccia, E., Turco, F., Palumbo, I., Lu, J., Steardo, A., … Steardo, L. (2014). Palmitoylethanolamide improves colon inflammation through an enteric glia/toll like receptor 4-dependent PPAR-α activation. *Gut, 63*(8), 1300-12. doi:

10.1136/gutjnl-2013-305005

Esposito, G., Filippis, D., Cirillo, C., Iuvone, T., Capoccia, E., Scuderi, C., … Steardo, L. (2013). Cannabidiol in inflammatory bowel diseases: a brief overview. *Phytother Res, 27*(5), 633-6. doi: 10.1002/ptr.4781

Fallahi, F., Borran, S., Ashrafizadeh, M., Zarrabi, A., Pourhanifeh, M., Khaksary Mahabady, M., … Mirzaei H. (2012). Curcumin and inflammatory bowel diseases: From in vitro studies to clinical trials. *Mol Immunol, 130*, 20-30. doi: 10.1016/j.molimm.2020.11.016

Fasano, A. (2012). Leaky gut and autoimmune diseases. *Clin Rev Allergy Immunol, 42*(1), 71-8. doi: 10.1007/s12016-011-8291-x

Fields, M. & Lewis, C. (1997). Impaired endocrine and exocrine pancreatic functions in copper-deficient rats: the effect of gender. *J Am Coll Nutr, 16*(4), 346-51. doi: 10.1080/07315724.1997.10718696

Fransisca, Y., Small, D., Morrison, P., Spencer, M., Ball, A. & Jones, O. (2015). Assessment of arsenic in Australian grown and imported rice varieties on sale in Australia and potential links with irrigation practises and soil geochemistry. *Chemosphere, 138*, 1008-13. doi: 10.1016/j.chemosphere.2014.12.048

Freeman, H. (2016). Endocrine manifestations in celiac

disease. *World J Gastroenterol, 22*(38), 8472-8479. doi: 10.3748/wjg.v22.i38.8472

Fric, P. & Zavoral, M. (2003). The effect of non-pathogenic Escherichia coli in symptomatic uncomplicated diverticular disease of the colon. *Eur J Gastroenterol Hepatol, 15*(3), 313-5. doi: 10.1097/01.meg.0000049998.68425.e2

Fujikawa, Y., Tominaga, K., Tanaka, F., Kamata, N., Yamagami, H., Tanigawa T, ... Arakawa, T. (2017). Postprandial symptoms felt at the lower part of the epigastrium and a possible association of pancreatic exocrine dysfunction with the pathogenesis of functional dyspepsia. *Intern Med, 56*(13),1629-1635. doi: 10.2169/internalmedicine.56.8193

Fujita, T. & Sakurai, K. (1995). Efficacy of glutamine-enriched enteral nutrition in an experimental model of mucosal ulcerative colitis. *Br J Surg, 82*(6), 749-51. doi: 10.1002/bjs.1800820611

Fuss, J., Bindila, L., Wiedemann, K., Auer, M., Briken, P. & Biedermann, S. (2017). Masturbation to Orgasm Stimulates the Release of the Endocannabinoid 2-Arachidonoylglycerol in Humans. *J Sex Med, 14*(11), 1372-1379. doi: 10.1016/j.jsxm.2017.09.016

Gabbard, S., Lacy, B., Levine, G. & Crowell, M. (2014). The impact of alcohol consumption and cholecystectomy on small intestinal bacterial overgrowth. *Dig Dis Sci,59*(3), 638- 44. doi: 10.1007/s10620-013-2960-y

Gable, S. (2006). Macroscope: The toxicity of recreational drugs. *Scientific American, 94*(3), 206

Galli, M., Morelli, R., Casellato, A. & Perna, M. (1986). Retrobulbar optic neuritis in a patient with acute type B hepatitis. *J Neurol Sci, 72*(2-3), 195-200. doi: 10.1016/0022-510x(86)90007-9

García, A., Salas-Jara, M., Herrera, C. & González, C. (2014). Biofilm and Helicobacter pylori: from environment to human host. *World J Gastroenterol, 20*(19), 5632-8. doi: 10.3748/wjg.v20.i19.5632

Gerstein, H. & VanderMeulen, J. (1996). The relationship between cow's milk exposure and type 1 diabetes. *Diabet Med, 13*(1), 23-9. doi: 10.1002/(SICI)1096-9136(199601)13:1<23::AID-DIA4>3.0.CO;2-D

Gertsch, J., Pertwee, R. & Di Marzo, V. (2010). Phytocannabinoids beyond the cannabis plant - do they exist? *Br J Pharmacol, 160*(3), 523-9. doi: 10.1111/j.1476-5381.2010.00745.x

Gesterling, L., & Bradford, H. (2022). Cannabis use in pregnancy: A state of the science review. *J Midwifery Womens Health, 67*(3), 305-313. doi: 10.1111/jmwh.13293

Ghoshal, U., Shukla, R. & Ghoshal, U. (2017). Small Intestinal Bacterial overgrowth and irritable bowel syndrome: A bridge between functional organic dichotomy. *Gut Liver, 11*(2), 196-208. doi: 10.5009/gnl16126

Giacosa, A., Morazzoni, P., Bombardelli, E., Riva, A., Bianchi Porro, G. & Rondanelli, M. (2015). Can nausea and vomiting be treated with ginger extract? *Eur Rev Med Pharmacol Sci, 19*(7),1291-6

Gibson, G., Hutkins, R., Sanders, M., Prescott, S, Reimer, R., Salminen S., … Reid, G. (2017). Expert consensus document: The International Scientific Association for Probiotics and Prebiotics (ISAPP) consensus statement on the definition and scope of prebiotics. *Nat Rev Gastroenterol Hepatol, 14*(8), 491-502. doi: 10.1038/nrgastro.2017.75

Gionchetti, P., Rizzello, F., Morselli, C., Romagnoli, R., & Campieri, M. (2005). Management of inflammatory bowel disease: does rifaximin offer any promise? *Chemotherapy, 51* Suppl 1, 96-102. doi: 10.1159/000081995

Goggin, R., Jardeleza, C., Wormald, P. & Vreugde, S. (2014) Colloidal silver: a novel treatment for Staphylococcus aureus biofilms? *Int Forum Allergy Rhinol,* 4(3), 171-5. doi: 10.1002/alr.21259

Gomez, R., Nichoalds, G., Singh, M., Simsek, H. &

LaSure, M. (1988). In vitro assay of pancreatic acinar-cell function of rats made chronically riboflavin deficient. *Am J Clin Nutr, 48*(3), 626-31. doi: 10.1093/ajcn/48.3.626

Graziani, G., Como, G., Badalamenti, S., Finazzi, S., Malesci, A., Gallieni, M., ... Ponticelli, C. (1995). Effect of gastric acid secretion on intestinal phosphate and calcium absorption in normal subjects. *Nephrol Dial Transplant, 10*(8), 1376-80)

Guo, Q., Goldenberg, J., Humphrey, C., El Dib, R. & Johnston, B. (2019). Probiotics for the prevention of pediatric antibiotic-associated diarrhea. *Cochrane Database of Systematic Reviews*, (4), CD004827. doi: 10.1002/14651858.CD004827.pub5

Guslandi, M. (2005). Antibiotics for inflammatory bowel disease: do they work? *Eur J Gastroenterol Hepatol, 17*(2), 145-7. doi: 10.1097/00042737-200502000-00003

Guslandi, M., Giollo, P. & Testoni, P. (2003). A pilot trial of Saccharomyces boulardii in ulcerative colitis. *Eur J Gastroenterol Hepatol, 15*(6), 697-8. doi: 10.1097/00042737-200306000-00017

Guslandi, M., Mezzi, G., Sorghi, M. & Testoni, P. (2000). Saccharomyces boulardii in maintenance treatment of Crohn's disease. *Dig Dis Sci, 45*(7), 1462-4. doi: 10.1023/a:1005588911207

Hadjivassiliou, M., Boscolo, S., Davies-Jones, G., Grünewald, R., Not, T., Sanders, D., ... Woodroofe, N. (2002). The humoral response in the pathogenesis of gluten ataxia. *Neurology, 58*(8), 1221-6. doi: 10.1212/wnl.58.8.1221

Hafström, I., Ringertz, B., Spångberg, A., von Zweigbergk, L., Brannemark, S., Nylander I, ... Klareskog, L. (2001). A vegan diet free of gluten improves the signs and symptoms of rheumatoid arthritis: the effects on arthritis correlate with a reduction in antibodies to food antigens. *Rheumatology (Oxford), 40*(10), 1175-9. doi: 10.1093/rheumatology/40.10.1175

Han, M., Anderson, R., Viennois, E. & Merlin, D. (2020). Examination of food consumption in United States adults and the prevalence of inflammatory bowel disease using National Health Interview Survey 2015. *PLoS One, 15*(4), e0232157. doi: 10.1371/journal.pone.0232157

Hansen, S., Melby, K., Aase, S., Jellum, E. & Vollset, S. (1999). Helicobacter pylori infection and risk of cardia cancer and non-cardia gastric cancer. A nested case-control study. *Scand J Gastroenterol, 34*(4), 353-60. doi: 10.1080/003655299750026353

Hardt, P., Krauss, A., Bretz, L., Porsch-Ozcürümez, M., Schnell-Kretschmer, H., Mäser, E., ... Klör, H. (2000).

Pancreatic exocrine function in patients with type 1 and type 2 diabetes mellitus. *Acta Diabetol, 37*(3), 105-10. doi: 10.1007/s005920070011

Harris, P., Serrano, C., Villagrán, A., Walker, M., Thomson, M., Duarte, I., … Crabtree, J. (2013). Helicobacter pylori-associated hypochlorhydria in children, and development of iron deficiency. *J Clin Pathol, 66*(4), 343-7. doi: 10.1136/jclinpath-2012-201243

Harris, P., Serrano, C., Villagrán, A., Walker, M., Thomson, M., Duarte, I., … Crabtree, J. (2013). Helicobacter pylori-associated hypochlorhydria in children, and development of iron deficiency. *J Clin Pathol, 66*(4), 343-7. doi: 10.1136/jclinpath-2012-201243

Hashiesh, H., Sharma, C., Goyal, S., Sadek, B., Jha, N., Kaabi, J. &, Ojha, S. (2021). A focused review on CB2 receptor-selective pharmacological properties and therapeutic potential of β-caryophyllene, a dietary cannabinoid. *Biomed Pharmacother, 140*, 111639. doi: 10.1016/j.biopha.2021.111639

Hernández-Lahoz, C. & Rodrigo, L. (2013). Trastornos relacionados con el gluten y enfermedades desmielinizantes [Gluten-related disorders and demyelinating diseases]. *Med Clin (Barc), 140*(7), 314-9. Spanish. doi: 10.1016/j.medcli.2012.07.009

Hijos-Mallada, G., Sostres, C. & Gomollón, F. (2022). NSAIDs, gastrointestinal toxicity and inflammatory bowel disease. *Gastroenterol Hepatol, 45*(3):215-222. English, Spanish. doi: 10.1016/j.gastrohep.2021.06.003

Hill, I., Fasano, A., Schwartz, R., Counts, D., Glock, M. & Horvath, K. (2000). The prevalence of celiac disease in at-risk groups of children in the United States. *J Pediatr, 136*(1), 86-90. doi: 10.1016/s0022-3476(00)90055-6

Ho, S., Woodford, K., Kukuljan, S. & Pal, S. (2014). Comparative effects of A1 versus A2 beta-casein on gastrointestinal measures: a blinded randomised cross-over pilot study. *Eur J Clin Nutr, 68*(9), 994-1000. doi: 10.1038/ejcn.2014.127

Hoffman, L., D'Argenio, D., MacCoss, M., Zhang, Z., Jones, R. & Miller, S. (2005). Aminoglycoside antibiotics induce bacterial biofilm formation. *Nature, 436*(7054), 1171-5. doi: 10.1038/nature03912

Holtmann, G., Kriebel, R. & Singer, M. (1990). Mental stress and gastric acid secretion. Do personality traits influence the response? *Dig Dis Sci, 35*(8), 998-1007. doi: 10.1007/BF01537249

Holzer, P. (2007) Taste receptors in the gastrointestinal tract. V. Acid sensing in the gastrointestinal tract. *Am J Physiol Gastrointest Liver Physiol, 292*(3):G699-705. doi: 10.1152/ajpgi.00517.2006

Homan, M. & Orel, R. (2015). Are probiotics useful in Helicobacter pylori eradication? *World J Gastroenterol, 21*(37), 10644-53. doi: 10.3748/wjg.v21.i37.10644

Huebner, F., Lieberman, K., Rubino, R. & Wall, J. (1984). Demonstration of high opioid-like activity in isolated peptides from wheat gluten hydrolysates. *Peptides, 5*(6), 1139-47. doi: 10.1016/0196-9781(84)90180-3

Iacono, G., Cavataio, F., Montalto, G., Florena, A., Tumminello, M., Soresi, M., … Carroccio, A. (1998). Intolerance of cow's milk and chronic constipation in children. *N Engl J Med, 339*(16), 1100-4. doi: 10.1056/NEJM199810153391602

Iñiguez, C., Mauri, J., Larrodé, P., López del Val, J., Jericó, I., & Morales, F. (2000). Mielitis transversa aguda secundaria a la vacunación de la hepatitis B [Acute transverse myelitis secondary to hepatitis B vaccination]. *Rev Neurol, 31*(5), 430-2. Spanish.

Isaacs, K. & Sartor, R. (2004). Treatment of inflammatory bowel disease with antibiotics. *Gastroenterol Clin North Am, 33*(2), 335-45, x. doi: 10.1016/j.gtc.2004.02.006

Ivarsson, A., Hernell, O., Stenlund, H. & Persson, L. (2002). Breast-feeding protects against celiac disease. *Am J Clin Nutr, 75*(5), 914-21. doi: 10.1093/ajcn/75.5.914

Ivarsson, A., Persson, L., Nyström, L. & Hernell, O. (2003). The Swedish coeliac disease epidemic with a prevailing twofold higher risk in girls compared to boys may reflect gender specific risk factors. *Eur J Epidemiol, 18*(7), 677-84. doi: 10.1023/a:1024873630588

Jakobsen, T., van Gennip, M., Phipps, R., Shanmugham, M., Christensen, L., Alhede, M., ... Givskov M. (2012). Ajoene, a sulfur-rich molecule from garlic, inhibits genes controlled by quorum sensing. *Antimicrob Agents Chemother, 56*(5):2314-25. doi: 10.1128/AAC.05919-11

Jarosz, M., Dzieniszewski, J., Dabrowska-Ufniarz, E., Wartanowicz, M., Ziemlanski, S. & Reed, P. (1998). Effects of high dose vitamin C treatment on Helicobacter pylori infection and total vitamin C concentration in gastric juice. *Eur J Cancer Prev, 7*(6):449-54. doi: 10.1097/00008469-199812000-00004

Jefferson, K. (2004). What drives bacteria to produce a biofilm? *FEMS Microbiol Lett, 236*(2), 163-73. doi: 10.1016/j.femsle.2004.06.005

Jiang, C., Li, G., Huang, P., Liu, Z. & Zhao, B. (2017). The gut microbiota and Alzheimer's disease. *J Alzheimers Dis, 58*(1), 1-15. doi: 10.3233/JAD-161141

Jianqin, S., Leiming, X., Lu, X., Yelland, G., Ni, J. & Clarke, A. (2016). Erratum to: 'Effects of milk containing only A2 beta casein versus milk containing both A1 and A2 beta casein proteins on gastrointestinal physiology, symptoms of discomfort, and cognitive behavior of people with self-reported intolerance to traditional cows' milk'. *Nutr J, 15*(1):45. doi: 10.1186/s12937-016-0164-y. Erratum for: *Nutr J, 15*:35. doi: 10.1186/s12937-016-0147-z

Jiménez, E., Fernández, L., Marín, M., Martín, R., Odriozola, J., Nueno-Palop, C., … Rodríguez, J. (2005). Isolation of commensal bacteria from umbilical cord blood of healthy neonates born by cesarean section. *Curr Microbiol, 51*(4), 270-4. doi: 10.1007/s00284-005-0020-3

Jiménez, E., Marín, M., Martín, R., Odriozola, J., Olivares, M., Xaus, J., … Rodríguez, J. (2008). Is meconium from healthy newborns actually sterile? *Res Microbiol, 159*(3), 187-93. doi: 10.1016/j.resmic.2007.12.007

Kahrs, C., Chuda, K., Tapia, G., Stene, L., Mårild, K., Rasmussen, T, … Størdal, K. (2019). Enterovirus as trigger of coeliac disease: nested case-control study within prospective birth cohort. *BMJ, 364*, l231. doi: 10.1136/bmj.l231

Kamaeva, O., Reznikov, IuP., Pimenova, N &, Dobritsyna, L. (1998). Antigliadinovye antitela v otsutstvie tseliakii [Antigliadin antibodies in the absence of celiac disease]. *Klin Med (Mosk), 76*(2), 33-5. Russian.

Kanauchi, O., Serizawa, I., Araki, Y., Suzuki, A., Andoh, A., Fujiyama, Y., ... Bamba, T. (2003). Germinated barley foodstuff, a prebiotic product, ameliorates inflammation of colitis through modulation of the enteric environment. *J Gastroenterol, 38*(2), 134-41. doi: 10.1007/s005350300022

Kang, D., Adams, J., Coleman, D., Pollard, E., Maldonado, J., McDonough-Means, S., ... Krajmalnik-Brown, R. (2019). Long-term benefit of microbiota transfer therapy on autism symptoms and gut microbiota. *Sci Rep, 9*(1), 5821. doi: 10.1038/s41598-019-42183-0

Kaplan, J. (2011). Antibiotic-induced biofilm formation. *Int J Artif Organs, 34*(9), 737-51. doi: 10.5301/ijao.5000027

Kasarda, D. (2013). Can an increase in celiac disease be attributed to an increase in the gluten content of wheat as a consequence of wheat breeding? *J Agric Food Chem, 61*(6), 1155-9. doi: 10.1021/jf305122s

Kato, S., Fujimura, S., Udagawa, H., Shimizu, T., Maisawa, S., Ozawa, K. & Iinuma, K. (2002). Antibiotic resistance of Helicobacter pylori strains in Japanese children. *J Clin Microbiol, 40*(2), 649-53. doi: 10.1128/JCM.40.2.649-653.2002

Kaye, M. (1979). On the relationship between gastric pH and pressure in the normal human lower oesophageal sphincter. *Gut, 20*(1), 59-63. doi: 10.1136/gut.20.1.59

Kelly, D. & Wischmeyer, P. (2003). Role of L-glutamine in critical illness: new insights. *Curr Opin Clin Nutr Metab Care, 6*(2), 217-22. doi: 10.1097/00075197-200303000-00011

Khademi, Z., Milajerdi, A., Larijani, B. & Esmaillzadeh, A. (2021). Dietary intake of total carbohydrates, sugar and sugar-sweetened beverages, and risk of inflammatory bowel disease: A systematic review and meta-analysis of prospective cohort studies. *Front Nutr, 8*, 707795. doi: 10.3389/fnut.2021.707795

Khan, M., Zahin, M., Hasan, S., Husain, F. & Ahmad, I. (2009). Inhibition of quorum sensing regulated bacterial functions by plant essential oils with special reference to clove oil. *Lett Appl Microbiol, 49*(3), 354-60. doi: 10.1111/j.1472-765X.2009.02666.x

Kim, D., Paik, C., Kim, Y., Lee, J., Jun, K., Chung, W., … Choi, M. (2017). Positive glucose breath tests in patients with hysterectomy, gastrectomy, and cholecystectomy. *Gut Liver, 11*(2), 237-242. doi: 10.5009/gnl16132

Kim, D., Paik, C., Song, D., Kim, Y. & Lee, J. (2018). The characteristics of small intestinal bacterial overgrowth in patients with gallstone diseases. *J Gastroenterol Hepatol, 33*(8), 1477-1484. doi: 10.1111/jgh.14113

Kirby, T. & Ochoa-Repáraz, J. (2018). The gut microbiome in multiple sclerosis: A potential therapeutic avenue. *Med Sci (Basel), 6*(3),69. doi: 10.3390/medsci6030069

Klein, C. , Hill, M., Chang, S., Hillard, C. & Gorzalka, B. (2012). Circulating endocannabinoid concentrations and sexual arousal in women. *J Sex Med.* 9(6):1588-601. doi: 10.1111/j.1743-6109.2012.02708.x

Kolokotroni, Middleton, Gavatha, Lamnisos, Priftis, & Yiallouros, (2012). Asthma and atopy in children born by caesarean section: effect modification by family history of allergies - a population based cross-sectional study. *BMC Pediatr, 12*, 179. doi: 10.1186/1471-2431-12-179

Korpela, K., Salonen, A., Virta, L., Kumpu, M., Kekkonen, R. & de Vos, W. (2016). Lactobacillus rhamnosus GG intake modifies preschool children's intestinal microbiota, alleviates penicillin-associated changes, and reduces antibiotic use. *PLoS One, 11*(4), e0154012. doi: 10.1371/journal.pone.0154012

Korzenik, J. (2006). Case closed? Diverticulitis: epidemiology and fiber. *J Clin Gastroenterol, 40 Suppl 3*, S112-6. doi: 10.1097/01.mcg.0000225503.59923.6c

Krott, L., Piscitelli, F., Heine, M., Borrino, S., Scheja, L., Silvestri, C., … Di Marzo, V. (2016). Endocannabinoid regulation in white and brown adipose tissue following thermogenic activation. *J Lipid Res,* 57(3), 464-73. doi: 10.1194/jlr.M065227

Kruis, W., Fric, P., Pokrotnieks, J., Lukás, M., Fixa, B., Kascák, M., … Schulze, J. (2004). Maintaining remission of ulcerative colitis with the probiotic Escherichia coli Nissle 1917 is as effective as with standard mesalazine. *Gut, 53*(11), 1617-23. doi: 10.1136/gut.2003.037747

Kukreja, A., & Maclaren, N. (2000). Current cases in which epitope mimicry is considered as a component cause of autoimmune disease: immune-mediated (type 1) diabetes. *Cell Mol Life Sci, 57*(4), 534-41. doi: 10.1007/PL00000715

Kwak, S., Robinson, S., Lee, J., Lim, H., Wallace, C. & Jin, Y. (2022). Dissection and enhancement of prebiotic properties of yeast cell wall oligosaccharides through metabolic engineering. *Biomaterials, 282*, 121379. doi: 10.1016/j.biomaterials.2022.121379

Kwieciński, J., Eick, S. & Wójcik. K. (2009). Effects of tea tree (Melaleuca alternifolia) oil on Staphylococcus aureus in biofilms and stationary growth phase. *Int J Antimicrob Agents, 33*(4), 343-7. doi: 10.1016/j.ijantimicag.2008.08.028

Lachenmeier, D. & Rehm, J. (2015). Comparative risk assessment of alcohol, tobacco, cannabis and other illicit drugs using the margin of exposure approach. *Sci Rep, 5*, 8126. doi: 10.1038/srep08126

Lane, E., Zisman, T. & Suskind, D. (2017). The microbiota in inflammatory bowel disease: current and therapeutic insights. *J Inflamm Res, 10*, 63-73. doi: 10.2147/JIR.S116088

Langmead, L., Feakins, R., Goldthorpe, S., Holt, H., Tsironi, E., De Silva, A., … Rampton, D. (2004). Randomized, double-blind, placebo-controlled trial of oral aloe vera gel for active ulcerative colitis. *Aliment Pharmacol Ther, 19*(7), 739-47. doi: 10.1111/j.1365-2036.2004.01902.x

Langmead, L., Dawson, C., Hawkins, C., Banna, N., Loo, S. & Rampton D. (2002). Antioxidant effects of herbal therapies used by patients with inflammatory bowel disease: an in vitro study. *Aliment Pharmacol Ther, 16*(2), 197-205. doi: 10.1046/j.1365-2036.2002.01157.x

LaPlante, K., Sarkisian, S., Woodmansee, S., Rowley, D. & Seeram, N. (2012). Effects of cranberry extracts on growth and biofilm production of Escherichia coli and Staphylococcus species. *Phytother Res, 26*(9), 1371-4. doi: 10.1002/ptr.4592

Lee, J., Kim, Y. & Lee, J. (2017). Carvacrol-rich oregano oil and thymol-rich thyme red oil inhibit biofilm formation and the virulence of uropathogenic Escherichia coli. *J Appl Microbiol, 123*(6), 1420-1428. doi: 10.1111/jam.13602

Lee, W., Yoon, W., Shin, H., Jeon, S. & Rhee P. (2008). Helicobacter pylori infection and motor fluctuations in patients with Parkinson's disease. *Mov Disord, 23*(12), 1696-700. doi: 10.1002/mds.22190

Lete, I. & Allué.J. (2016). The effectiveness of ginger in the prevention of nausea and vomiting during pregnancy and chemotherapy. *Integr Med Insights, 11*,11-7. doi: 10.4137/IMI.S36273

Leventogiannis, K., Gkolfakis, P., Spithakis, G., Tsatali, A., Pistiki, A., Sioulas, A., … Triantafyllou, K. (2019). Effect of a preparation of four probiotics on symptoms of patients with irritable bowel syndrome: Association with intestinal bacterial overgrowth. *Probiotics Antimicrob Proteins, 11*(2), 627-634. doi: 10.1007/s12602-018-9401-3

Lewis, S. & Heaton, K. (1997). Stool form scale as a useful guide to intestinal transit time. *Scand J Gastroenterol, 32*(9), 920-4. doi: 10.3109/00365529709011203

Li, H., He, T., Xu, Q., Li, Z., Liu Y, Li, F., … Liu, C. (2015). Acupuncture and regulation of gastrointestinal function. *World J Gastroenterol, 21*(27), 8304-13. doi: 10.3748/wjg.v21.i27.8304

Li, Q., Han, Y., Dy, A. & Hagerman, R. (2017). The gut microbiota and autism spectrum disorders. *Front Cell Neurosci, 11*, 120. doi: 10.3389/fncel.2017.00120

Ligresti, A., Villano, R., Allarà, M., Ujváry, I. & Di Marzo, V. (2012). Kavalactones and the endocannabinoid system: the plant-derived yangonin is a novel CB_1 receptor ligand. *Pharmacol Res, 66*(2),163-9. doi: 10.1016/j.phrs.2012.04.003

Lionetti, E., Castellaneta, S., Francavilla, R., Pulvirenti, A., Tonutti, E., Amarri, S., … Catassi C; SIGENP (Italian Society of Pediatric Gastroenterology, Hepatology, and Nutrition) (2014). Working group on weaning and CD risk. Introduction of gluten, HLA status, and the risk of celiac disease in children. *N Engl J Med, 371*(14), 1295-303. doi: 10.1056/NEJMoa1400697

Liu, B., Fang, F., Pedersen, N., Tillander, A., Ludvigsson, J., Ekbom, A., … Wirdefeldt K. (2017). Vagotomy and Parkinson disease: A Swedish register-based matched-cohort study. *Neurology, 88*(21),1996-2002. doi: 10.1212/WNL.0000000000003961

Liu, Y. & Forsythe, P. (2021). Vagotomy and insights

into the microbiota-gut-brain axis. *Neurosci Res,168*, 20-27. doi: 10.1016/j.neures.2021.04.001

Liu, Z. & Udenigwe, C. (2019). Role of food-derived opioid peptides in the central nervous and gastrointestinal systems. *J Food Biochem, 43*(1), e12629. doi: 10.1111/jfbc.12629

Lombardo, L., Foti, M., Ruggia, O. & Chiecchio, A. (2010). Increased incidence of small intestinal bacterial overgrowth during proton pump inhibitor therapy. *Clin Gastroenterol Hepatol, 8*(6):504-8. doi: 10.1016/j.cgh.2009.12.022

Ludvigsson, J. & Green, P. (2014). The missing environmental factor in celiac disease. *N Engl J Med, 371*(14). 1341-3. doi: 10.1056/NEJMe1408011

Luna, R., Savidge, T. & Williams, K. (2016). The brain-gut-microbiome axis: What role does it play in autism spectrum disorder? *Curr Dev Disord Rep, 3*(1), 75-81. doi: 10.1007/s40474-016-0077-7

Lynch, S. & Boushey, H. (2016). The microbiome and development of allergic disease. *Curr Opin Allergy Clin Immunol,16*(2), 165- 71. doi: 10.1097/ACI.0000000000000255

Mahady, G., Pendland, S., Yun, G. & Lu, Z. (2002). Turmeric (Curcuma longa) and curcumin inhibit the growth of Helicobacter pylori, a group 1 carcinogen.

Anticancer Res, 22(6C), 4179-81

Maintz, L. & Novak, N. (2007). Histamine and histamine intolerance. *Am J Clin Nutr, 85*(5), 1185-96. doi: 10.1093/ajcn/85.5.1185

Makipour, K. & Friedenberg, F. (2011). The potential role of N-acetylcysteine for the treatment of Helicobacter pylori. *J Clin Gastroenterol, 45*(10), 841-3. doi: 10.1097/MCG.0b013e31822be4d6

Makkawi. S., Camara-Lemarroy, C. & Metz, L. (2018). Fecal microbiota transplantation associated with 10 years of stability in a patient with SPMS. *Neurol Neuroimmunol Neuroinflamm, 5*(4), e459. doi: 10.1212/NXI.0000000000000459

Malchow, H. (1997). Crohn's disease and Escherichia coli. A new approach in therapy to maintain remission of colonic Crohn's disease? *J Clin Gastroenterol, 25*(4), 653-8. doi: 10.1097/00004836-199712000-00021

Manousos, O., Day, N., Tzonou, A., Papadimitriou, C., Kapetanakis, A., Polychronopoulou-Trichopoulou, A. & Trichopoulos, D. (1985). Diet and other factors in the aetiology of diverticulosis: an epidemiological study in Greece. *Gut, 26*(6), 544-9. doi: 10.1136/gut.26.6.544

Marton, L., Goulart, R., Carvalho, A. & Barbalho, S. (2019). Omega fatty acids and inflammatory bowel diseases: An overview. *Int J Mol Sci, 20*(19), 4851. doi:

10.3390/ijms20194851

Maruvada, P., Leone, V., Kaplan, L. & Chang, E. (2017). The human microbiome and obesity: Moving beyond associations. *Cell Host Microbe, 22*(5), 589-599. doi: 10.1016/j.chom.2017.10.005

McAllister, S., Soroceanu L. & Desprez, P. (2015). The Antitumor Activity of Plant-Derived Non-Psychoactive Cannabinoids. *J Neuroimmune Pharmacol, 10*(2), 255-67. doi: 10.1007/s11481-015-9608-y

McDougle, D., Watson, J., Abdeen, A., Adili, R., Caputo, M., Krapf, J., … Das, A. (2017). Anti-inflammatory ω-3 endocannabinoid epoxides. *Proc Natl Acad Sci U S A, 114*(30), E6034-E6043. doi: 10.1073/pnas.1610325114

McGee, D., Lu, X., & Disbrow, E. (2018). Stomaching the possibility of a pathogenic role for Helicobacter pylori in Parkinson's disease. *J Parkinsons Dis, 8*(3), 367-374. doi: 10.3233/JPD-181327

Metyas, S., Chen, C., Yeter, K., Solyman, J. & Arkfeld, D. (2018). Low dose naltrexone in the treatment of fibromyalgia. *Curr Rheumatol Rev, 14*(2), 177-180. doi: 10.2174/1573397113666170321120329

Mollenbrink, M. & Bruckschen, E. (1994). Behandlung der chronischen obstipation mit physiologischen Escherichia-coli-Bakterien. Med Klin, 89, 587-93.

Montgomery, R., Haboubi, N., Mike, N., Chesner, I. & Asquith, P. (1986). Causes of malabsorption in the elderly. *Age Ageing, 15*(4),235-40. doi: 10.1093/ageing/15.4.235

Moré, M. & Swidsinski, A. (2015). Saccharomyces boulardii CNCM I-745 supports regeneration of the intestinal microbiota after diarrheic dysbiosis - a review. *Clin Exp Gastroenterol, 8*, 237-55. doi: 10.2147/CEG.S85574

Mulle, J., Sharp, W. & Cubells, J. (2013). The gut microbiome: a new frontier in autism research. *Curr Psychiatry Rep, 15*(2), 337. doi: 10.1007/s11920-012-0337-0

Murtagh J. (1992). Diarrhoea. *Aust Fam Physician, 21*(5), 668-9, 672-3.

Myléus, A., Hernell, O., Gothefors, L., Hammarström, M., Persson, L., Stenlund, H. & Ivarsson, A. (2012). Early infections are associated with increased risk for celiac disease: an incident case-referent study. *BMC Pediatr, 12*, 194. doi: 10.1186/1471-2431-12-194

Nguyen, L., Örtqvist, A., Cao, Y., Simon, T., Roelstraete, B., Song, M., … Ludvigsson J. (2020). Antibiotic use and the development of inflammatory bowel disease: a national case-control study in Sweden.

Lancet Gastroenterol Hepatol, 5(11), 986-995. doi: 10.1016/S2468-1253(20)30267-3

Nunes, A., Pontes, J., Rosa, A., Gomes, L., Carvalheiro, M. & Freitas, D. (2003). Screening for pancreatic exocrine insufficiency in patients with diabetes mellitus. *Am J Gastroenterol, 98*(12), 2672-5. doi: 10.1111/j.1572-0241.2003.08730.x

Ozutemiz, A., Aydin, H., Isler, M., Celik, H. & Batur, Y. (2002). Effect of omeprazole on plasma zinc levels after oral zinc administration. *Indian J Gastroenterol, 21*(6), 216-8.

Pandit, S., Ravikumar, V., Abdel-Haleem, A., Derouiche, A., Mokkapati, V., Sihlbom, C., … Mijakovic, I. (2017). Low concentrations of vitamin C reduce the synthesis of extracellular polymers and destabilize bacterial biofilms. *Front Microbiol, 8*, 2599. doi: 10.3389/fmicb.2017.02599

Paray, B., Albeshr, M., Jan, A., & Rather I. (2020). Leaky gut and autoimmunity: An intricate balance in individuals health and the diseased state. *Int J Mol Sci, 21*(24), 9770. doi: 10.3390/ijms21249770

Parker, L., Rock, E. & Limebeer, C. (2011). Regulation of nausea and vomiting by cannabinoids. *Br J Pharmacol, 163*(7):1411-22. doi: 10.1111/j.1476-5381.2010.01176.x.

Passani, M., Panula, P. & Lin, J. (2014). Histamine in the brain. *Front Syst Neurosci, 8*, 64. doi: 10.3389/fnsys.2014.00064

Patten, D., Schultz, B. & Berlau, D. (2018). The safety and efficacy of low-dose naltrexone in the management of chronic pain and inflammation in multiple sclerosis, fibromyalgia, Crohn's disease, and other chronic pain disorders. *Pharmacotherapy, 38*(3), 382-389. doi: 10.1002/phar.2086

Pérez-Maceda, B., López-Bote, J., Langa, C. & Bernabeu, C. (1991). Antibodies to dietary antigens in rheumatoid arthritis--possible molecular mimicry mechanism. *Clin Chim Acta, 203*(2-3), 153-65. doi: 10.1016/0009-8981(91)90287-m

Perisetti, A., Gajendran, M., Dasari, C., Bansal, P., Aziz, M., Inamdar, S., … Goyal, H. (2020). Cannabis hyperemesis syndrome: an update on the pathophysiology and management. *Ann Gastroenterol, 33*(6):571-578. doi: 10.20524/aog.2020.0528

Persson, P., Ahlbom, A. & Hellers, G. (1992). Diet and inflammatory bowel disease: a case-control study. *Epidemiology, 3*(1), 47-52. doi: 10.1097/00001648-199201000-00009

Peterson, C., Sharma, V., Uchitel, S., Denniston, K., Chopra, D., Mills, P. & Peterson, S. (2018). Prebiotic potential of herbal medicines used in digestive health and disease. *J Altern Complement Med, 24*(7), 656-665. doi: 10.1089/acm.2017.0422

Pierantozzi, M., Pietroiusti, A., Sancesario, G., Lunardi, G., Fedele, E., Giacomini, P., …Stanzione, P. (2001). Reduced L-dopa absorption and increased clinical fluctuations in Helicobacter pylori-infected Parkinson's disease patients. *Neurol Sci, 22*(1), 89-91. doi: 10.1007/s100720170061

Pointer, S., Rickstrew, J., Slaughter, J., Vaezi, M., & Silver H. (2016). Dietary carbohydrate intake, insulin resistance and gastro-oesophageal reflux disease: a pilot study in European- and African-American obese women. *Aliment Pharmacol Ther, 44*(9), 976-988. doi: 10.1111/apt.13784

Prantera, C., Scribano, M., Falasco, G., Andreoli, A. & Luzi, C. (2002). Ineffectiveness of probiotics in preventing recurrence after curative resection for Crohn's disease: a randomised controlled trial with Lactobacillus GG. *Gut, 51*(3), 405-9. doi: 10.1136/gut.51.3.405

Pruimboom, L. & de Punder, K. (2015). The opioid effects of gluten exorphins: asymptomatic celiac disease. *J Health Popul Nutr, 33*, 24. doi: 10.1186/s41043-015-0032-y

Pugin, B., Barcik, W., Westermann, P., Heider, A., Wawrzyniak, M., Hellings, P., … O'Mahony, L.

(2017). A wide diversity of bacteria from the human gut produces and degrades biogenic amines. *Microb Ecol Health Dis, 28*(1), 1353881. doi: 10.1080/16512235.2017.1353881

Pulikkan, J., Mazumder, A. & Grace, T. (2019). Role of the gut microbiome in autism spectrum disorders. *Adv Exp Med Biol,* 1118, 253-269. doi: 10.1007/978-3-030-05542-4_13

Racine, A., Carbonnel, F., Chan, S., Hart, A., Bueno-de-Mesquita, H., Oldenburg, B., ... Boutron-Ruault, M. (2016). Dietary patterns and risk of inflammatory bowel disease in Europe: Results from the EPIC study. *Inflamm Bowel Dis, 22*(2), 345-54. doi: 10.1097/MIB.0000000000000638

Rahman, M., Rahman, M., Reichman, S., Lim, R. & Naidu, R. (2014). Arsenic speciation in Australian-grown and imported rice on sale in Australia: implications for human health risk. *J Agric Food Chem, 62*(25), 6016-24. doi: 10.1021/jf501077w

Randal Bollinger, R., Barbas, A., Bush, E., Lin, S. & Parker, W. (2007). Biofilms in the large bowel suggest an apparent function of the human vermiform appendix. *J Theor Biol, 249*(4), 826-31. doi: 10.1016/j.jtbi.2007.08.032

Rao, S. & Brenner, D. (2021). Efficacy and safety of over-the-counter therapies for chronic constipation: An updated systematic review. *Am J Gastroenterol, 116*(6), 1156-1181. doi: 10.14309/ajg.0000000000001222

Rappaport, E. (1955). Achlorhydria; associated symptoms and response to hydrochloric acid. *N Engl J Med, 252*(19), 802-5. doi: 10.1056/NEJM195505122521904

Reddavide, R., Rotolo, O., Caruso, M., Stasi, E., Notarnicola, M., Miraglia, C., … Leandro, G. (2018). The role of diet in the prevention and treatment of Inflammatory Bowel Diseases. *Acta Biomed, 89*(9-S), 60-75. doi: 10.23750/abm.v89i9-S.7952

Reif, S., Klein, I., Lubin, F., Farbstein, M., Hallak, A. & Gilat, T. (1997). Pre-illness dietary factors in inflammatory bowel disease. *Gut, 40*(6), 754-60. doi: 10.1136/gut.40.6.754

Rezaie, A., Buresi, M., Lembo, A., Lin, H., McCallum, R., Rao, S., … Pimentel, M. (2017). Hydrogen and methane-based breath testing in gastrointestinal disorders: The North American consensus. *Am J Gastroenterol, 112*(5), 775-784. doi: 10.1038/ajg.2017.46

Ried, K., Travica, N., Dorairaj, R. & Sali, A. (2020). Herbal formula improves upper and lower gastrointestinal symptoms and gut health in Australian adults with digestive disorders. *Nutr Res, 76*, 37-51. doi: 10.1016/j.nutres.2020.02.008

Rodakis, J. (2015). An n=1 case report of a child with autism improving on antibiotics and a father's quest to understand what it may mean. *Microb Ecol Health Dis, 26*, 26382. doi: 10.3402/mehd.v26.26382

Rodrigo, L., Hernandez-Lahoz, C., Fuentes, D., Mauri, G., Alvarez, N., Vega J.,& Gonzalez, S. (2014). Randomised clinical trial comparing the efficacy of a gluten-free diet versus a regular diet in a series of relapsing-remitting multiple sclerosis patients. *Int J Neurol Neurother, 1*, 012. doi: 10.23937/2378-3001/1/1/1012

Rojas, M., Restrepo-Jiménez, P., Monsalve, D., Pacheco, Y., Acosta-Ampudia, Y., Ramírez-Santana, C., … Anaya J. (2018). Molecular mimicry and autoimmunity. *J Autoimmun, 95*, 100-123. doi: 10.1016/j.jaut.2018.10.012

Roland, B., Ciarleglio, M., Clarke, J., Semler, J., Tomakin, E., Mullin, G. & Pasricha, P. (2014). Low ileocecal valve pressure is significantly associated with small intestinal bacterial overgrowth (SIBO). *Dig Dis Sci, 59*(6), 1269-77. doi: 10.1007/s10620-014-3166-7

Rosenblatt, J., Reitzel, R., Vargas-Cruz, N., Chaftari, A., Hachem, R. & Raad, I. (2017). Caprylic and polygalacturonic acid combinations for eradication of microbial organisms embedded in biofilm. *Front Microbiol, 8*, 1999. doi: 10.3389/fmicb.2017.01999

Rostenberg, A. (2018). Your Genius Body, Publ. Red Mountain Natural Medicine ISBN-13 9780578393261

Rothenbacher, D., Löw, M., Hardt, P., Klör, H., Ziegler, H. & Brenner, H. (2005). Prevalence and determinants of exocrine pancreatic insufficiency among older adults: results of a population-based study. *Scand J Gastroenterol, 40*(6), 697-704. doi: 10.1080/00365520510023116

Rousseaux, C., Thuru, X., Gelot, A., Barnich, N., Neut, C., Dubuquoy, L., … Desreumaux, P. (2007). Lactobacillus acidophilus modulates intestinal pain and induces opioid and cannabinoid receptors. *Nat Med, 13*(1), 35-7. doi: 10.1038/nm1521

Ruscin, J., Page, R., 2nd, & Valuck, R. (2002). Vitamin B(12) deficiency associated with histamine(2)-receptor antagonists and a proton-pump inhibitor. *Ann Pharmacother, 36*(5), 812-6. doi: 10.1345/aph.10325

Russell, R. (1997). Gastric hypochlorhydria and achlorhydria in older adults. *JAMA, 278*(20),1659.doi:10.1001/jama.1997.03550200035022

Ruyssers, N., De Winter, B., De Man, J., Loukas, A., Herman, A., Pelckmans, P. & Moreels, T. (2008). Worms and the treatment of inflammatory bowel disease: are molecules the answer? *Clin Dev Immunol, 2008*, 567314. doi: 10.1155/2008/567314

Ryan, J., Heckler, C., Roscoe, J., Dakhil, S., Kirshner, J., Flynn, P., ... Morrow, G. (2012). Ginger (Zingiber officinale) reduces acute chemotherapy-induced nausea: a URCC CCOP study of 576 patients. *Support Care Cancer, 20*(7), 1479-89. doi: 10.1007/s00520-011-1236-3

Sałaga, M., Sobczak, M. & Fichna, J. (2014). Inhibition of fatty acid amide hydrolase (FAAH) as a novel therapeutic strategy in the treatment of pain and inflammatory diseases in the gastrointestinal tract. *Eur J Pharm Sci, 52*, 173-9. doi: 10.1016/j.ejps.2013.11.012

Salminen, P., Paajanen, H., Rautio, T., Nordström, P., Aarnio, M., Rantanen, T., ... Grönroos, J. (2015). Antibiotic therapy vs appendectomy for treatment of uncomplicated acute appendicitis: The APPAC Randomized Clinical Trial. *JAMA, 313*(23), 2340-8. doi: 10.1001/jama.2015.6154

Sampson, T., Debelius, J., Thron, T., Janssen, S., Shastri, G., Ilhan, Z., ... Mazmanian S. (2016). Gut microbiota regulate motor deficits and neuroinflammation in a model of Parkinson's disease. *Cell, 167*(6), 1469-1480.e12. doi: 10.1016/j.cell.2016.11.018

Sandler, R., Finegold, S., Bolte, E., Buchanan, C., Maxwell, A., Väisänen, M., ... Wexler, H. (2000). Short-term benefit from oral vancomycin treatment of regressive-onset autism. *J Child Neurol, 15*(7),429-35. doi: 10.1177/088307380001500701

Santelmann, H., Laerum, E., Roennevig, J. & Fagertun, H. (2001). Effectiveness of nystatin in polysymptomatic patients. A randomized, double-blind trial with nystatin versus placebo in general practice. *Fam Pract, 18*(3), 258-65. doi: 10.1093/fampra/18.3.258\

Santos-García, D., Arias-Rivas, S., Dapena, D. & Arias, M. (2007). Infección remota por virus de la hepatitis B y enfermedad desmielinizante multifásica: ¿casualidad o causalidad? [Past hepatitis B virus infection and demyelinating multiphasic disease: casual or causal relationship?]. *Neurologia, 22*(8), 542-6. Spanish.

Sarnelli, G., D'Alessandro, A., Iuvone, T., Capoccia, E., Gigli, S., Pesce, M., … Esposito, G. (2016). Palmitoylethanolamide modulates inflammation-associated vascular endothelial growth factor (VEGF) signaling via the Akt/mTOR pathway in a selective peroxisome proliferator-activated receptor alpha (PPAR-α)-dependent manner. *PLoS One, 11*(5), e0156198. doi: 10.1371/journal.pone.0156198

Saukkonen, T., Virtanen, S., Karppinen, M., Reijonen, H., Ilonen, J., Räsänen, L., … Savilahti, E. (1998). Significance of cow's milk protein antibodies as risk factor for childhood IDDM: interactions with dietary cow's milk intake and HLA-DQB1 genotype. Childhood Diabetes in Finland Study Group. *Diabetologia, 41*(1), 72-8. doi: 10.1007/s001250050869

Scheperjans, F., Aho, V., Pereira, P., Koskinen, K., Paulin, L., Pekkonen, E., ... Auvinen P. (2015). Gut microbiota are related to Parkinson's disease and clinical phenotype. *Mov Disord, 30*(3), 350-8. doi: 10.1002/mds.26069

Schicho, R. & Storr, M. (2014). Cannabis finds its way into treatment of Crohn's disease. *Pharmacology, 93*(1-2), 1-3. doi: 10.1159/000356512

Schneider, A., Streitberger, K. & Joos, S. (2007). Acupuncture treatment in gastrointestinal diseases: a systematic review. *World J Gastroenterol, 13*(25), 3417-24. doi: 10.3748/wjg.v13.i25.3417

Segal, Y. & Shoenfeld, Y. (2018). Vaccine-induced autoimmunity: the role of molecular mimicry and immune crossreaction. *Cell Mol Immunol, 15*(6), 586-594. doi: 10.1038/cmi.2017.151

Seidner, D., Lashner, B., Brzezinski, A., Banks, P., Goldblum, J., Fiocchi, C., ... Demichele, S. (2005). An oral supplement enriched with fish oil, soluble fiber, and antioxidants for corticosteroid sparing in ulcerative colitis: a randomized, controlled trial. *Clin Gastroenterol Hepatol, 3*(4), 358-69. doi:

10.1016/s1542-3565(04)00672-x

Seo, M., Okada, M., Yao, T., Furukawa, H. & Matake, H. (1999). The role of total parenteral nutrition in the management of patients with acute attacks of inflammatory bowel disease. *J Clin Gastroenterol, 29*(3), 270-5. doi: 10.1097/00004836-199910000-00009

Shay, H & Gershan-Cohen J. (1936). A comparison of the effectiveness of glutamic acid hydrochloride and dilute hydrochloric acid as the replacement therapy in acidity measured by fractional gastric acid titration and hydrogen-ion concentration curves. *Ann Int Med, 9,* 1628-1638

Sheaffer, K., Kim, R., Aoki, R., Elliott, E., Schug, J., Burger, L., … Kaestner, K. (2014). DNA methylation is required for the control of stem cell differentiation in the small intestine. *Genes Dev, 28*(6), 652-64. doi: 10.1101/gad.230318.113

Shiraishi, T. (1988). Hypothalamic control of gastric acid secretion. *Brain Res Bull, 20*(6), 791-7. doi: 10.1016/0361-9230(88)90093-7

Shor, D., Barzilai, O., Ram, M., Izhaky, D., Porat-Katz, B., Chapman, J., … Shoenfeld, Y. (2009). Gluten sensitivity in multiple sclerosis: experimental myth or clinical truth? *Ann N Y Acad Sci, 1173*, 343-9. doi: 10.1111/j.1749-6632.2009.04620.x

Sidebotham, R., Worku, M., Karim, Q., Dhir, N. & Baron J. (2003). How Helicobacter pylori urease may affect external pH and influence growth and motility in the mucus environment: evidence from in-vitro studies. *Eur J Gastroenterol Hepatol, 15*(4), 395-401. doi: 10.1097/00042737-200304000-00010

Siguel, E. & Lerman, R. (1996). Prevalence of essential fatty acid deficiency in patients with chronic gastrointestinal disorders. *Metabolism, 45*(1), 12-23. doi: 10.1016/s0026-0495(96)90194-8

Sikander, A., Rana, S. & Prasad, K. (2009). Role of serotonin in gastrointestinal motility and irritable bowel syndrome. *Clin Chim Acta, 403*(1-2), 47-55. doi: 10.1016/j.cca.2009.01.028

Silverman, M., Davis, I. & Pillai, D. (2010). Success of self-administered home fecal transplantation for chronic Clostridium difficile infection. *Clin Gastroenterol Hepatol, 8*(5), 471-3. doi: 10.1016/j.cgh.2010.01.007

Simon, J., Hudes, E. & Perez-Perez, G. (2003). Relation of serum ascorbic acid to Helicobacter pylori serology in US adults: the Third National Health and Nutrition Examination Survey. *J Am Coll Nutr, 22*(4), 283-9. doi: 10.1080/07315724.2003.10719305

Singh, M. (1986). Effect of niacin and niacin-tryptophan deficiency on pancreatic acinar cell function in rats in vitro. *Am J Clin Nutr, 44*(4):512-8. doi: 10.1093/ajcn/44.4.512

Singh, R., Chang, H., Yan, D., Lee, K., Ucmak, D., Wong, K., ... Liao, W. (2017). Influence of diet on the gut microbiome and implications for human health. *J Transl Med, 15*(1), 73. doi: 10.1186/s12967-017-1175-y

Sivam, G. (2001). Protection against Helicobacter pylori and other bacterial infections by garlic. *J Nutr, 131*(3s):1106S-8S. doi: 10.1093/jn/131.3.1106S

Sjöstedt, P., Enander, J. & Isung, J. (2021). Serotonin reuptake inhibitors and the gut microbiome: Significance of the gut microbiome in relation to mechanism of action, treatment response, side effects, and tachyphylaxis. *Front Psychiatry, 12*, 682868. doi: 10.3389/fpsyt.2021.682868

Smith, C., Crowther, C. & Beilby, J. (2002). Acupuncture to treat nausea and vomiting in early pregnancy: a randomized controlled trial. *Birth, 29*(1),1-9. doi: 10.1046/j.1523-536x.2002.00149.x

Smith, G. & Pell, J (2003). Parachute use to prevent death and major trauma related to gravitational challenge: systemic review of randomised trials. *BMJ, 327,* 1459. doi:10.1136/bmj.327.7429.1459

Smith, L., Azariah, F., Lavender, V., Stoner, N. &

Bettiol, S. (2015). Cannabinoids for nausea and vomiting in adults with cancer receiving chemotherapy. *Cochrane Database Syst Rev, 2015*(11), CD009464. doi: 10.1002/14651858.CD009464.pub2

Smith, R., Talley, N., Dent, O., Jones, M. & Waller, S. (1991). Exocrine pancreatic function and chronic unexplained dyspepsia. A case-control study. *Int J Pancreatol, 8*(3), 253-62. doi: 10.1007/BF02924544

Smolka, A. & Schubert, M. (2017). Helicobacter pylori-induced changes in gastric acid secretion and upper gastrointestinal disease. *Curr Top Microbiol Immunol, 400*, 227-252. doi: 10.1007/978-3-319-50520-6_10

Smyk, D., Koutsoumpas, A., Mytilinaiou, M., Rigopoulou, E., Sakkas, L. & Bogdanos, D. (2014). Helicobacter pylori and autoimmune disease: cause or bystander. *World J Gastroenterol, 20*(3), 613-29. doi: 10.3748/wjg.v20.i3.613

Sonnenborn, U. & Schulze, J. (2009). The non-pathogenic *Escherichia coli* strain Nissle 1917 – features of a versatile probiotic. *Microbial Ecology in Health and Disease, 21*(3-4),122-158, doi:10.3109/08910600903444267

Sonnenburg, J. & Sonnenburg, E (2015). Gut feelings– the "second brain" in our gastrointestinal systems. *Scientific American* 1 May 2015

Sparling, P., Giuffrida, A., Piomelli, D., Rosskopf, L. & Dietrich, A. (2003). Exercise activates the endocannabinoid system. *Neuroreport, 14*(17), 2209-11. doi: 10.1097/00001756-200312020-00015

Spencer, N., Hibberd, T., Travis, L., Wiklendt, L., Costa, M., Hu, H., … Sorensen J. (2018). Identification of a rhythmic firing pattern in the enteric nervous system that generates rhythmic electrical activity in smooth muscle. *J Neurosci, 38*(24), 5507-5522. doi: 10.1523/JNEUROSCI.3489-17.2018

Sreevalsan, S., Joseph, S., Jutooru, I., Chadalapaka, G. & Safe, S. (2011). Induction of apoptosis by cannabinoids in prostate and colon cancer cells is phosphatase dependent. *Anticancer Res, 31*(11), 3799-807

Staley, C., Hamilton, M., Vaughn, B., Graiziger, C., Newman, K., Kabage, A., … Khoruts, A. (2017). Successful resolution of recurrent Clostridium difficile infection using freeze-dried, encapsulated fecal microbiota; Pragmatic Cohort Study. *Am J Gastroenterol, 112*(6), 940-947. doi: 10.1038/ajg.2017.6

Stermer, E., Tabak, M., Potasman, I., Levy, N., Tamir, A. & Neeman, I. (1997). Effect of ranitidine on the urea breath test: a controlled trial. *J Clin Gastroenterol, 25*(1), 323-7. doi: 10.1097/00004836-199707000-

00005

Storr, M. & Sharkey, K. (2007). The endocannabinoid system and gut-brain signalling. *Curr Opin Pharmacol,* *7*(6), 575-82. doi: 10.1016/j.coph.2007.08.008

Strate, L., Liu, Y., Aldoori, W. & Giovannucci, E. (2009). Physical activity decreases diverticular complications. *Am J Gastroenterol, 104*(5), 1221-30. doi: 10.1038/ajg.2009.121

Strate, L., Liu, Y., Aldoori, W., Syngal, S. & Giovannucci, E. (2009). Obesity increases the risks of diverticulitis and diverticular bleeding. *Gastroenterology, 136*(1), 115-122.e1. doi: 10.1053/j.gastro.2008.09.025

Strate, L., Liu, Y., Huang, E., Giovannucci, E. & Chan A. (2011). Use of aspirin or nonsteroidal anti-inflammatory drugs increases risk for diverticulitis and diverticular bleeding. *Gastroenterology, 140*(5), 1427-33. doi: 10.1053/j.gastro.2011.02.004

Sturniolo, G, Di Leo, V., Ferronato, A., D'Odorico, A., & D'Incà, R. (2001). Zinc supplementation tightens "leaky gut" in Crohn's disease. *Inflamm Bowel Dis, 7*(2), 94-8. doi: 10.1097/00054725-200105000-00003

Sturniolo, G., Montino, M., Rossetto, L., Martin, A., D'Inca, R., D'Odorico, A., Naccarato, R. (1991). Inhibition of gastric acid secretion reduces zinc absorption in man. *J Am Coll Nutr, 10*(4), 372-5. doi: 10.1080/07315724.1991.10718165

Summers, R., Elliott, D., Urban, J. Jr, Thompson, R. & Weinstock, J. (2005). Trichuris suis therapy in Crohn's disease. *Gut, 54*(1), 87-90. doi: 10.1136/gut.2004.041749

Summers, R., Elliott, D., Urban, J. Jr, Thompson, R. & Weinstock, J. (2005). Trichuris suis therapy for active ulcerative colitis: a randomized controlled trial. *Gastroenterology, 128*(4), 825-32. doi: 10.1053/j.gastro.2005.01.005

Sung, H., Paik, C., Chung, W., Lee, K., Yang, J. & Choi, M. (2015). Small intestinal bacterial overgrowth diagnosed by glucose hydrogen breath test in post-cholecystectomy patients. *J Neurogastroenterol Motil, 21*(4),545-51. doi: 10.5056/jnm15020

Takahashi, T. (2006). Acupuncture for functional gastrointestinal disorders. *J Gastroenterol, 41*(5), 408-17. doi: 10.1007/s00535-006-1773-6

Takahashi, S., Igarashi, H., Masubuchi, N., Ishiyama, N., Saito, S., Aoyagi, T., … Hirata, I. (1993). [Helicobacter pylori and the development of atrophic gastritis]. *Nihon Rinsho, 51*(12), 3231-5. Japanese.

Targownik, L., Lix, L., Metge, C., Prior, H., Leung, S.

& Leslie, W. (2008). Use of proton pump inhibitors and risk of osteoporosis-related fractures. *CMAJ, 179*(4), 319-26. doi: 10.1503/cmaj.071330

Tayarani-Najaran, Z., Talasaz-Firoozi, E., Nasiri, R., Jalali, N. & Hassanzadeh, M. (2013). Antiemetic activity of volatile oil from Mentha spicata and Mentha × piperita in chemotherapy-induced nausea and vomiting. *Ecancermedicalscience, 7*, 290. doi: 10.3332/ecancer.2013.290

Termanini, B., Gibril, F., Sutliff, V., Yu, F., Venzon, D. & Jensen, T. (1998). Effect of long-term gastric acid suppressive therapy on serum vitamin B12 levels in patients with Zollinger-Ellison syndrome. *Am J Med, 104(*5), 422-30. doi: 10.1016/s0002-9343(98)00087-4

Thiéfin, G. & Beaugerie, L. (2005). Toxic effects of nonsteroidal antiinflammatory drugs on the small bowel, colon, and rectum. *Joint Bone Spine, 72*(4), 286-94. doi: 10.1016/j.jbspin.2004.10.004

Tsujikawa, T., Satoh, J., Uda, K., Ihara, T., Okamoto, T., Araki, Y., ... Bamba, T. (2000). Clinical importance of n-3 fatty acid-rich diet and nutritional education for the maintenance of remission in Crohn's disease. *J Gastroenterol. 2000;35*(2):99-104. doi: 10.1007/s005350050021

Turunen, P., Wikström, H., Carpelan-Holmström, M., Kairaluoma, P., Kruuna, O. & Scheinin, T. (2010). Smoking increases the incidence of complicated diverticular disease of the sigmoid colon. *Scand J Surg, 99*(1), 14-7. doi: 10.1177/145749691009900104

Uemura, N., Okamoto, S., Yamamoto, S., Matsumura, N., Yamaguchi, S., Yamakido, M., ... Schlemper, R. (2001). Helicobacter pylori infection and the development of gastric cancer. *N Engl J Med, 345*(11), 784-9. doi: 10.1056/NEJMoa001999

Ul Haq, M. (2020). Gluten Exorphins. In: Opioid Food Peptides. Springer, Singapore. https://doi.org/10.1007/978-981-15-6102-3_6

van den Broeck, H., de Jong, H., Salentijn, E., Dekking, L., Bosch, D., Hamer, R., ... Smulders, M. (2010). Presence of celiac disease epitopes in modern and old hexaploid wheat varieties: wheat breeding may have contributed to increased prevalence of celiac disease. *Theor Appl Genet, 121*(8), 1527-39. doi: 10.1007/s00122-010-1408-4

Vaona, B., Stanzial, A., Talamini, G., Bovo, P., Corrocher, R. & Cavallini, G. (2005). Serum selenium concentrations in chronic pancreatitis and controls. *Dig Liver Dis, 37*(7), 522-5. doi: 10.1016/j.dld.2005.01.013

Vaughn, A., Haas, K., Burney, W., Andersen, E., Clark, A., Crawford, R. & Sivamani, R. (2017). Potential role of curcumin against biofilm-producing organisms on the skin: A review. *Phytother Res, 31*(12):1807-1816. doi: 10.1002/ptr.5912

Villumsen, M., Aznar, S., Pakkenberg, B., Jess, T. & Brudek, T. (2019). Inflammatory bowel disease increases the risk of Parkinson's disease: a Danish nationwide cohort study 1977-2014. *Gut, 68*(1), 18-24. doi: 10.1136/gutjnl-2017-315666

Virtanen, S., Saukkonen, T., Savilahti, E., Ylönen, K., Räsänen, L., Aro, A., ... Akerblom, H. (1994). Diet, cow's milk protein antibodies and the risk of IDDM in Finnish children. Childhood Diabetes in Finland Study Group. *Diabetologia, 37*(4), 381-7. doi: 10.1007/s001250050121

Vreugdenhil, G., Geluk, A., Ottenhoff, T., Melchers, W., Roep, B. & Galama, J. (1998). Molecular mimicry in diabetes mellitus: the homologous domain in coxsackie B virus protein 2C and islet autoantigen GAD65 is highly conserved in the coxsackie B-like enteroviruses and binds to the diabetes associated HLA-DR3 molecule. *Diabetologia, 41*(1), 40-6. doi: 10.1007/s001250050864

Walter, J. (2008). Ecological role of lactobacilli in the gastrointestinal tract: implications for fundamental and biomedical research. *Appl Environ Microbiol, 74*(16), 4985-96. doi: 10.1128/AEM.00753-08

Wang, K., Li, S., Liu, C., Perng, D., Su, Y., Wu, D., … Wang W. (2004). Effects of ingesting Lactobacillus- and Bifidobacterium-containing yogurt in subjects with colonized Helicobacter pylori. *Am J Clin Nutr, 80*(3), 737-41. doi: 10.1093/ajcn/80.3.737

Wang, Z., Li, H., Kang, Y., Liu, Y., Shan, L. & Wang, F. (2022). Risks of digestive system side-effects of selective serotonin reuptake inhibitors in patients with depression: A network meta-analysis. *Ther Clin Risk Manag, 18*, 799-812. doi: 10.2147/TCRM.S363404

Wanke, C. (2001). Do probiotics prevent childhood illnesses? *BMJ, 322*(7298), 1318-9. doi: 10.1136/bmj.322.7298.1318

Wapnir, R. (2000). Zinc deficiency, malnutrition and the gastrointestinal tract. *J Nutr, 30*(5S Suppl), 1388S-92S. doi: 10.1093/jn/130.5.1388S

Weaver, K. & Herfarth, H. (2021). Gluten-free diet in IBD: Time for a recommendation? *Mol Nutr Food Res, 65*(5):e1901274. doi: 10.1002/mnfr.201901274

Williams, P. (2009). Incident diverticular disease is inversely related to vigorous physical activity. *Med Sci Sports Exerc, 41*(5), 1042-7. doi: 10.1249/MSS.0b013e318192d02d

Willis, K., Purvis, J., Myers, E., Aziz, M., Karabayir, I., Gomes, C., … Pierre, J. (2019). Fungi form interkingdom microbial communities in the primordial human gut that develop with gestational age. *FASEB J, 33*(11), 12825-12837. doi: 10.1096/fj.201901436RR

Wollin, A., Wang, X. & Tso, P. (1998). Nutrients regulate diamine oxidase release from intestinal mucosa. *Am J Physiol, 275*(4), R969-75. doi: 10.1152/ajpregu.1998.275.4.R969

Yadav, D. & Pitchumoni, C. (2003). Issues in hyperlipidemic pancreatitis. *J Clin Gastroenterol, 36*(1), 54-62. doi: 10.1097/00004836-200301000-00016

Yancy, W. Jr., Provenzale, D. & Westman, E. (2001). Improvement of gastroesophageal reflux disease after initiation of a low-carbohydrate diet: five brief case reports. *Altern Ther Health Med, 7*(6), 120, 116-9.

Yano J., Yu, K., Donaldson, G., Shastri, G., Ann, P., Ma L., … Hsiao, E. (2015). Indigenous bacteria from the gut microbiota regulate host serotonin biosynthesis. *Cell, 161*(2), 264-76. doi: 10.1016/j.cell.2015.02.047

Yavari Kia, P., Safajou, F., Shahnazi, M. & Nazemiyeh, H. (2014). The effect of lemon inhalation aromatherapy on nausea and vomiting of pregnancy: a double-blinded, randomized, controlled clinical trial. *Iran Red Crescent Med J, 16*(3), e14360. doi: 10.5812/ircmj.14360

Yimam, K., Merriman, R. & Todd Frederick, R. (2013). A rare case of acute hepatitis B virus infection causing guillain-barré syndrome. *Gastroenterol Hepatol (N Y), 9*(2), 121-3.

Yin, H., Chu, A., Li, W., Wang, B., Shelton, F., Otero, F., ... Chen, Y. (2009). Lipid G protein-coupled receptor ligand identification using beta-arrestin PathHunter assay. *J Biol Chem, 284*(18), 12328-38. doi: 10.1074/jbc.M806516200

Young, D., Morton, R, & Bartley, J. (2010). Therapeutic ultrasound as treatment for chronic rhinosinusitis: preliminary observations. *J Laryngol Otol, 124*(5), 495-9. doi: 10.1017/S0022215109992519

Younger, J., Parkitny, L. & McLain, D. (2014). The use of low-dose naltrexone (LDN) as a novel anti-inflammatory treatment for chronic pain. *Clin Rheumatol, 33*(4), 451-9. doi: 10.1007/s10067-014-2517-2

Yuksel, F., Karatug, N. & Akcelik, M. (2018). Does subinhibitory concentrations of clinically important antibiotic induce biofilm production of Enterococcus faecium strains? *Acta Microbiol Immunol Hung, 65*(1), 27-38. doi: 10.1556/030.64.2017.041

Zhang, C., Li, Z., Pan, Q., Fan, L., Pan, T., Zhu, F., ... Zhao, L. (2022). Berberine at sub-inhibitory concentration inhibits biofilm dispersal in *Staphylococcus aureus. Microbiology (Reading), 168*(9). doi: 10.1099/mic.0.001243

Zhang, H., Feng, X., Larssen, T., Qiu, G. & Vogt, R. (2010). In inland China, rice, rather than fish, is the major pathway for methylmercury exposure. *Environ Health Perspect, 118*(9), 1183-8. doi: 10.1289/ehp.1001915

Zhou, G., Shi, Q., Huang, X. & Xie, X. (2015). The Three Bacterial Lines of Defense against Antimicrobial Agents. *Int J Mol Sci, 16*(9), 21711-33. doi: 10.3390/ijms160921711

Zhou, H., Jia, W., Liao, Y., Retnakaran, R., Krewski, D., Wen, S., … He, Y. (2023) Effects of vaginal microbiota transfer on the neurodevelopment and microbiome of cesarean-born infants: A blinded randomized controlled trial. *Cell Host Microbe. 231*(7):1232-1247.e5. doi: 10.1016/j.chom.2023.05.022

Zhou, Q., Verne, M., Fields, J., Lefante, J., Basra, S., Salameh, H. & Verne, G. (2019). Randomised placebo-controlled trial of dietary glutamine supplements for postinfectious irritable bowel syndrome. *Gut, 68*(6), 996-1002. doi: 10.1136/gutjnl-2017-315136

Żółkiewicz, J., Marzec, A., Ruszczyński, M., & Feleszko, W. (2020). Postbiotics-A Step Beyond Pre- and Probiotics. *Nutrients, 12*(8), 2189. doi: 10.3390/nu12082189